Disclosure in Health and Illness

Disclosure is a frequently used but rarely interrogated concept in health and social welfare. Abuse, disability, sexuality and health status can be 'disclosed' to peers and professionals and, on some occasions, disclosure is a requirement and not a choice. This innovative collection examines the new social and political implications of disclosure practices in health and illness.

We make our identities and our connections with others by sharing life stories, experiences and innermost desires, and are often asked to disclose facts about our lives, bodies and minds, at times with unintended consequences. Yet how and what, why and when people 'disclose' – and perceive, question and expose – and in what ways, has rarely received critical analytic attention. The contributors take up these problems by foregrounding the many shades of disclosure: from the secret, through the telling of diagnosis, to the more prosaic sharing of narratives from everyday life. The processes and implications of disclosing are addressed in areas such as: illness trajectories and end-of-life decisions; ethical research practices; medical procedures; and interpersonal relationships.

Exploring the idea of disclosure as a moral imperative and a social act, this book offers a diverse range of empirical case studies, social theories and methodological insights to show how dominant and normative understandings of social relationships and their obligations shape our understanding of acts of disclosure, enquiry and exposure. It will be of interest to students and academics with an interest in narrative studies, medical anthropology, bioethics, health psychology, health studies and the sociology of health and illness.

Mark Davis is Senior Lecturer in the School of Political and Social Inquiry at Monash University, Australia.

Lenore Manderson is Professor in the School of Public Health, University of the Witwatersrand, South Africa. She was formerly Professor of Medical Anthropology at Monash University, Australia, and is editor of the international journal, *Medical Anthropology*.

Routledge Studies in the Sociology of Health and Illness

Available titles include:

Dimensions of Pain
Humanities and Social Science Perspectives
Edited by Lisa Folkmarson Käll

Caring and Well-being
A Lifeworld Approach
Kathleen Galvin and Les Todres

Aging Men, Masculinities and Modern Medicine
Edited by Antje Kampf, Barbara L. Marshall and Alan Petersen

Disclosure in Health and Illness
Edited by Mark Davis and Lenore Manderson

Forthcoming titles:

Domestic Violence in Diverse Contexts
A Re-examination of Gender
Sarah Wendt and Lana Zannettino

The Public Shaping of Medical Research
Patient Associations, Health Movements and Biomedicine
Edited by Peter Wehling and Willy Viehöver

Abuse, Mental Illness and Recovery in Everyday Lives
Beyond Trauma
Nicole Moulding

Disclosure in Health and Illness

Edited by
**Mark Davis and
Lenore Manderson**

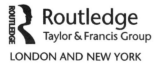

Routledge
Taylor & Francis Group

LONDON AND NEW YORK

First published 2014 by Routledge

2 Park Square, Milton Park, Abingdon, Oxfordshire OX14 4RN
52 Vanderbilt Avenue, New York, NY 10017

Routledge is an imprint of the Taylor & Francis Group, an informa business

First issued in paperback 2019

British Library Cataloguing in Publication Data
A catalogue record for this book is available from the British Library

Library of Congress Cataloging in Publication Data
Disclosure in health and illness/edited by Mark Davis and
   Lenore Manderson.
   pages cm
   1. Medical records – Access control. 2. Confidential
   communications – Access control. 3. Disclosure of information
   – Social aspects. 4. Privacy, Right of. I. Davis, Mark, 1963
   March 1– editor of compilation. II. Manderson, Lenore, editor
   of compilation.
   RC564.D57 2014
   651.5'04261 – dc23
   2013038351

ISBN: 978-0-415-70247-8 (hbk)
ISBN: 978-0-367-34139-8 (pbk)

Typeset in Sabon
by Florence Production Ltd, Stoodleigh, Devon, UK

Contents

Contributors

Janet Boddy is Reader in Child, Youth and Family Studies and Co-Director of the Centre for Innovation and Research in Childhood and Youth at the University of Sussex (www.sussex.ac.uk/esw/circy). Her interest in cross-national research with children and families includes studies of mainstream and targeted services, and recent publications include a chapter in *Family Troubles* (2013) on European approaches to family support.

Carole H. Browner is Distinguished Research Professor in the UCLA Semel Institute for Neuroscience and Human Behavior, the Department of Anthropology and the Department of Gender Studies. She has published widely on the social impact of decoding the human genome, including, with H. Mabel Preloran, *Neurogenetic Diagnoses: The Power of Hope and the Limits of Today's Medicine* (2010).

Mark Davis is Senior Lecturer at the School of Political and Social Inquiry, Monash University, Australia. His research addresses the technological mediation of intimate life and public health. His publications include *Sex, Technology and Public Health* (2009) and *HIV Treatment and Prevention Technologies in International Perspective*, edited with Corinne Squire (2010).

Devin Flaherty is a graduate student in UCLA's Department of Anthropology, where she studies medical and psychological anthropology with a special interest in death and dying. She received her MA from UCLA in 2013.

Paul Flowers is Professor of Sexual Health Psychology at Glasgow Caledonian University. He is interested in how the social sciences can contribute to applied health research and its influence on policy development. His own research focuses upon mixed methods and sexual health promotion. He is a Trustee of the National AIDS Trust.

Renata Kokanovic is Associate Professor at the School of Political and Social Inquiry, Monash University, Australia. Her research explores the socio-cultural context for subjective experiences of mental distress. She has published extensively, including her recent chapter in the *Sage Handbook of Mental Illness*, 'The diagnosis of depression in an international context' (2011).

Lenore Manderson is Professor in the School of Public Health, University of the Witwatersrand, South Africa. She was formerly Professor of Medical Anthropology at Monash University, Australia, and is editor of the international journal, *Medical Anthropology*. Her research is concerned with chronic illness, gender and sexuality, migration and inequality. Her recent publications include *Surface Tensions: Surgery, Bodily Boundaries and the Social Self* (2011) and, as editor, *Technologies of Sexuality, Identity and Sexual Health* (2012).

Brigid Philip is Research Fellow at the School of Political and Social Inquiry, Monash University, Australia. Her research is concerned with depression, emotional distress, neuroscience, neoliberalism and gender. She has published in *The Sociology of Health and Illness* and the *Journal of Sociology*.

H. Mabel Preloran is Research Anthropologist at the UCLA NPI-Semel Institute for Neuroscience and Human Behavior. Her research focuses on medical and psychological anthropology in the contexts of social change. She is the co-author of *Neurogenetic Diagnoses: The Power of Hope and the Limits of Today's Medicine* (2010).

Robin Root is Associate Professor in the Department of Sociology and Anthropology at Baruch College, USA. Her research in Malaysia and Swaziland has focused on how ideologies of biomedicine and religion affect people's experiences of self and sickness. Her work has been published in journals of anthropology and public health.

Corinne Squire is Professor of Social Sciences and Co-Director of the Centre for Narrative Research, University of East London. Her research interests are in HIV and citizenship, popular culture and subjectivities, and narrative theory and methods. Her most recent publications include *Living with HIV and ARVs: Three-Letter Lives* (2013) and, as co-editor with Molly Andrews and Maria Tamboukou, *Doing Narrative Research* (2008 and 2013).

Muriel Vernon is Lecturer in the Department of Anthropology and a staff research assistant in the Department of Family Medicine at UCLA. Her research focuses on the social efficacy of biomedical interventions, HIV/AIDS and MSM populations, and on transgender health and culture.

Matthew Wolf-Meyer is Associate Professor of Anthropology at the University of California, Santa Cruz. His work focuses on medicine, science and media in the United States. His first book, *The Slumbering Masses* (2012), offers insight into the complex lived realities of disorderly sleepers, the long history of sleep science, and the global impacts of the exportation of American sleep.

1 Telling points

Lenore Manderson

Disclosure is about telling, in all meanings of the word. Telling is an act of narration, it is a revelation, and it is a reflection of the importance of the information so imparted; the telling in disclosure is therefore a noun, a verb and an adjective. The stories that are told in disclosure typically hold deep significance for the storyteller; they are neither mundane facts nor simple biographic details. For this reason, the telling is staged. How such telling occurs tells us much about the teller, the witness, and the social times in which such acts of disclosure take place, as well as of the secrets that are disclosed. Yet typically we speak of disclosure lightly, as Corinne Squire suggests (this volume), without questioning its content, form, or cultural salience. We rarely interrogate the nature of disclosure, or the ways in which telling is structured and institutionalised, mandated and manipulated. In this introductory chapter, I worry at the complexities of disclosure and telling, anticipating the rich empirical examples and analytic details provided in the chapters that follow.

The social imperatives of disclosure

Disclosure, and the cultural protocols that shape telling, are central to how we establish and maintain intimate relationships, learn of and address medical diagnoses, disease and dying, conduct research with other humans, and manage public life. In various official contractual settings, disclosure is mandatory: a person wishing to borrow money or access credit is obliged to reveal all financial encumbrances; applicants for life insurance must disclose preexisting health problems. Everyday acts of disclosure are underpinned by social conventions that draw upon ideas about truth and the importance of truth telling. Official documents, including birth and marriage certificates, passports and drivers' licences, are presumed to tell certain personal truths as much as demographic facts about the bearer, and given this, the production and possession of forged documents are indictable offences. But such documents are also technologies of disclosure and exposure. Consider sex, in this context, and the power of documentation for people who are transsexual (see Vernon, this volume). The letter of the law, its rule, and its processes centre on ideas of truth and truth telling, reinforced in court hearings through oath or pledge. Similarly, cultural ideas about the importance of truth telling and the right to know influence how private, secret or suppressed information is provided to and reported by journalists.

Disclosure shapes much of economic life too. Selling and purchasing anything from food or medication to a house or a car are underpinned by explicit disclosures, including statements that prove that an item can be sold or that the product is safe. Ideas about disclosure inform the law, and establish what people are required to do by law, and these ideas are echoed in ethical statements and practices, economic transactions, everyday inter-actions and interpersonal relationships.

In this volume we set aside considerations of politics, law and economics, and focus on health, illness and personal life. But it is important to note, at the outset, that ideas about telling and truth inform how people interact in all kinds of social contexts. Jurisdictions vary, even within one nation, with regard to the mandatory or volitional disclosure of being HIV positive prior to having sex, for instance, regardless of the decision around safe sex. Yet at the same time, in everyday life, truth telling is implicit and normative, and the word of the individual is often enough. While legally people who are HIV-positive cannot donate blood, semen, ova or any other body tissues, the means of disclosure, a statement on an application form, is usually sufficient. We assume that people introduce themselves in a truthful way, and we accept as truthful the disclosures that unfold in autobiographic accounts. Hence the distress for the person who has received and accepted such stories when the accounts unravel, and the disclosure is discovered or exposed to be confabulation, fraud, delusion or wilful misrepresentation.

The timing of telling

Because disclosure is a particular kind of telling (Flaherty, Pleloran and Browner, this volume), the construction of truth and how its telling unfolds is never a trivial matter. In intimate contexts, both small specific and larger more profound disclosures take place as private acts. The timing and intent of telling are also disclosures, often of expectation, trust and risk, and under-standings of intimacy and care. They illustrate how disclosure can occur in anticipation of changes in relationships, or reflect the perceived maturity of and evolving trust within a relationship.

Disclosure involves telling the truth of an aspect of the self – being HIV positive, for instance, or experiencing depression. This is so even if the teller resists the facts that are disclosed as revealing essential or fundamental truths, as suggested in this volume in relation to mental health status (Kokanovic and Philip) and natal sex (Vernon). Consequently, disclosure positions the discloser in relation to others (or one other, the disclosee); in this volume, these disclosures are often statements of biosociality, as illustrated in relation to HIV (see Davis and Flowers, Root, and Squire) and Huntington's disease (Flaherty, Pleloran and Browner). And by virtue of the need for another, the telling, although often treated as private, is also always a public fact.

The risks to telling the truth include rejection, discriminatory actions and physical violence, and hence people employ various strategies to disclose or conceal. Each decision about disclosure asks an individual to weigh up the costs of truth or its suppression, including the relevance of a truth to other interpersonal and social ties, acts and engagement. For instance, HIV may not be considered by a person to be an essential truth of the self, but telling (or not telling) is an aspect of the representation of self, and the context of telling can shape the receipt and interpretation of knowledge. Disclosure of a medical condition may be received as a warning of risk of infection, for instance, but it also or instead may be presented and interpreted as a statement of community identity and membership, or as a gesture of trust.

In deliberating on the nature of truth and the importance of disclosure, as revisited and elaborated in the following chapters, I wish to consider how a single statement to one other person about the bioself (disclosing HIV status, transsexuality, or living with depression, for instance) is only the beginning of a sequence of social acts and exchanges of information. Our understanding of this, as social researchers, reveals how disclosure features in social and political, private and public lives. With HIV, for example, disclosure has become a central act in negotiating intimate relationships, in light of understandings of the moral and public health responsibility (as opposed to the legal imperative) to tell (potential) partners of possible health risks or exposure to infection. These ideas extend variably to STIs such as chlamydia, HPV and HSV, and to other blood-borne viruses (e.g. HBV, HCV). Each of these disclosures – the presence of an infection – is also a disclosure by proxy of other personal culturally nuanced facts, such as a history of unprotected sex, possible multiple partners, possible injecting drug use.

Disclosure unfolds in many different ways, even in this contained example of HIV. This includes the decision that must be made to tell or not to tell of HIV status in the context of an imminent or anticipated sexually intimate encounter. The disclosure may occur through a speech act, itself a simple statement of infection status or an extended revelatory explanation of sexual history and testing, or it may occur by proxy, by openly taking medication or reaching for a condom, for instance. These decisions of timing, form and content are framed by legal requirements, moral values, fear and expediency. Other HIV disclosures and concealments occur in the course of various mundane and strategic activities. They involve decision-making about whether and how to tell family members, friends, doctors and dentists, work colleagues, insurance companies, superannuation fund managers, and national governments (on applying for a visa, for instance) (see for instance Hardon and Posel 2012). The strategic concealments, in these contexts, are as important as the disclosures, and as self-conscious, as one example on the website of the Australian Federation of AIDS Organizations (AFAO) (2013) illustrates: 'I keep my HIV-pills in vitamin bottles. It avoids unplanned disclosure.' And, insofar as social life is always fluid and changing, as relationships evolve, this decision making about disclosure is also routinely revisited.

Even these examples limit our understanding of how and when disclosure occurs. Disclosure can be the unintended consequences of other actions or associations, as occurs for people with HIV who present to a health service established to meet their needs. Matthew Wilhelm-Solomon (2013) illustrates how in a displacement camp in northern Uganda, the provision and distribution of food aid and water containers, as well as antiretroviral therapy and other services, by association exposed some people to others in the camp as HIV-positive, in consequence producing HIV-specific health identities with ambiguous results. In this example, the different kinds of foods provided to people registered as HIV-positive (yellow soy beans rather than white maize), the days on which food parcels were delivered, and the colour of water containers (white not yellow) all indexed HIV positivity, 'transcending the paradigms of voluntary or involuntary disclosure' (Wilhelm-Solomon 2013: 232). Isak Niehaus similarly illustrates the cost of disclosure in relation to a person's HIV status. In his research setting, knowledge of HIV infection implied sexual promiscuity, so opening up speculation about others who might be infected, and precipitating social interactions based on ideas of the liminality of people with HIV, as living between life and death (Niehaus 2014).

Ashforth and Nattrass (2005: 293) draw attention to the power of these presumptions in shaping the decisions of people to disclose publicly, even for those who are in other ways outspoken activists, because of the possibility of discrimination including in health services, or because knowledge of another's HIV status might precipitate violent assault. Such public acts of abjection reinforce concerns about the risks of disclosing either volitionally or unintentionally (Tenkorang et al. 2011, Parle and Scorgie 2012, Scorgie et al. 2013). Since institutions, settings, bodies and technologies are not innocent, people who directly address whether or not to reveal a particular truth of the self must manage the flow of information to prevent the seepage of knowledge that might cause harm. Wilhelm-Solomon's examples of the discriminatory distribution of food aid and the colour-coding of water containers illustrate how easy it is to expose someone else, pre-empting their choice to disclose or not. Where knowledge has public currency of some kind, disclosures can occur through context, association and action, as well as explicit speech acts.

By way of a different example, Sargent and Kitobi (2012) write of the challenges faced by north African women living in Paris to control their fertility, and the strategies that they employ to disguise from their husbands and others their use of contraception. Accordingly, women hide contraceptive pills, or choose a method such as an injectable or an implant to avoid detection and possible consequent physical and verbal violence, abandonment, or polygamy, were they found to be using contraception without spousal permission. Yet even the most 'secret' methods may be discovered by a suspicious husband feeling for and discovering an implantable rod under the skin of his wife's upper arm, for instance, or by others, observing the woman's regular visits to a clinic and speculating on the causes of her doing so. Woman therefore regularly make difficult decisions as they negotiate fragile relationships which might implode in the face of disclosures of various histories of the body: sexual history, experience and preference, abortion, contraceptive use, sterilisation, sexually transmissible infections, HIV, or a history of sexual assault (see, for instance, de Zorda 2012).

Containing the truth

Because much is at stake when private information becomes public knowledge, people use complicated manoeuvres to contain disclosure and keep private facts secret. Any exposure or disclosure, whether orchestrated, unintended or circumstantial, impacts personally and interpersonally. Abortion is routinely concealed when it is procured, to avoid interference by the sexual partner responsible (or other partner), by family members, and, where its procurement is illegal, by the state and its representatives. But it is also concealed over the long term so that the woman can avoid disapprobation and unsolicited questions of honour (Shellenberg et al. 2011, van der Sijpt 2012, Astbury-Ward, Parry and Carnwell 2012). Further, negative attitudes to abortion impact health providers as well as clients (Harris et al. 2011, Youatt et al. 2012), for the stigma that is associated with certain actions, bodily histories and diseases routinely flows from the primary actor to others in their social world.

In a similar way, tuberculosis is 'risky' for the person infected, not only because of its infectious nature and severe morbidity, and the effects that this has on diagnosis and treatment (Murray et al. 2013), but also because of its symbolic and symptomatic links to HIV and the stigma and social marginalisation associated with both infections (Daftary 2012). Again, family members, health workers and others share this stigma. Further, because stigma extends to people working in occupations and industries most despised for cultural reasons (waste management, for instance), even a person's occupation may be withheld because of the social risks of disclosure. Ben Okri's award-winning novel *The Famished Road* (1991), and the account therein of the efforts that Azaro's father takes to avoid exposure to his family and community as a night soil collector, is a case in point. The idea of disclosure as impacting only or primarily on the speaker – the keeper of the secret – is therefore a very partial truth. The recipient of the truth disclosed is also affected, if only because telling cannot be revoked; the acts and facts of disclosure are indelible. This is true for both private and public disclosures which, as already indicated, reveal far more than a person's biostatus. Health-related disclosures, for example, routinely index other aspects of sexuality, sexual practices, drug-related behaviour, and so on. Further, while there is an illusion of relative equality when disclosures are made between the one who discloses and the one who receives the disclosure in intimate relationships of private actors, gender, age and other social structures destabilise presumed equality and sharpen concerns of what might be at stake in any disclosure. Differences in social and structural status trouble statements of the self.

The adoption of children provides a vivid example in this respect, partly because all people are affected by the decision (forced or voluntary) to surrender an infant to another person. In different jurisdictions, this act of surrender has changed significantly over a very short time, with changes to social attitudes and the state's accommodation of ex-nuptial births, as well as changes in laws that govern the right to adoption and access to personal information (e.g. the date and place of birth, the name of the mother, genetics and birthright). The formal apologies to women who were forced to give up children for adoption, which took place in 2013 in Australia, illustrate dramatic shifts in ideas about genetic origin and social parenting, and the scientific, social and economic policies that help shape these in the past fifty years. But they also rehearse the ethical and moral dilemmas and emotional weight of other reproductive decisions and possible disclosures – around surrogacy, gamete donation, and IVF (in vitro fertilisation), for example (van Berkell et al. 2007, Readings et al. 2011).

The stigma that makes disclosure a risk is explored in this volume particularly in relation to mental health problems (see chapters from Kokanovic and Philip, this volume; Seeman 2013) and sleep disorders (Wolf-Meyer, this volume). Because of the social and economic impact of a history of mental illness, or of sleepiness, consciousness and its productive importance, knowledge is managed at multiple levels. As both Kokanovic and Philip, and Wolf-Meyer illustrate, people very carefully weigh up the costs and benefits before speaking or acting. The high risk for parents with mental illness of losing their children (Hollingsworth, Swick and Choi 2013), temporarily or permanently through state intervention, suggests one reason behind the reluctance of people to seek mental health care and practical assistance, although the surveillance of parents by child protection agencies is compounded by other considerations. In the case of intimate partner violence, for instance, Rose and colleagues (2011) argue that people with mental health problems also fear that disclosure (of violence) would not be believed, compounding reasons that prevent reporting and ameliorative action in such circumstances (Westad and McConnell 2012).

Although disclosure is understood to be a statement of an important truth, how and when that truth is shared is subject to debate and circumstance, context and culture. The decision to disclose or withhold is always framed by interpersonal relationships and their value, since disclosure definitionally is a statement of the self to another (or others). It implies personal agency and, if this is true, then Wilhelm-Solomon's example of food aid and water containers is an instance of exposure rather than disclosure. One discloses one's self; others expose. But in addition, the private or quasi-private interpersonal nature of disclosure, as sketched out above in relation to HIV, is one small example of how we might understand telling. Since disclosure is about the self, the decision to disclose is richly imbued with questions of identity and relationality. As we illustrate, chronic non-communicable conditions, HIV, sexual health, inheritable diseases and mental illness provide us with case studies to consider methodological questions and substantive concerns, including the particularities and commonalities of different health states and communities. Further, our focus on health and illness allows us to develop theoretical understandings that translate readily to other domains. Sexual abuse, addiction, criminality, wealth, inheritance and family history all come to mind as personal fields that may be no less volatile than sexual history, infection or health status, or genetic risk. These matters of disclosure all evoke considerations around confidentiality, trust, risk, intimacy, and fear or its disposition.

Autobiographic and other personal information may be deemed worthy to tell as 'essential truths' of the teller, but also, as suggested in the case of HIV, because of the direct impact of the disclosed facts on the health and wellbeing of the other. In such cases, acts of disclosure and the ethical considerations that influence telling are reasonably clear. But we need to look more closely at other allied concepts and contexts to better understand disclosure as both a public and private act, and to link disclosure to related and distinctive concepts and actions, including those of truth, privacy, secrecy, exposure and closure. These are concepts all at the heart of much social (inter)action. In the process of such unpacking, disclosure takes us back to Foucault's world of biopolitics, power and knowledge (e.g. Foucault 1978). Differences in social and structural status, always apparent in clinical encounters but also in work settings, overdetermine who discloses what information, and at what cost.

Medical disclosures

Disclosure is a fundamental and underlying principle of clinical relationships, human bioethics and professional and institutional life. Disclosure is translated into a set of responsibilities in research practices, working environments and in clinical relationships, although what is disclosed, and by whom, is routinely subject to review. Disclosure by doctors to patients is incorporated into medical training, a central element in effective medical care despite shifts in guidelines and their practice. Disclosure is central to any discussion of the practice of medical diagnosis, treatment choices and regimes, and prognosis, and to the component parts of these sequences of events. Ideas of the cultural significance of disclosure of a diagnosis of cancer, for example, fold into disclosures of its prognosis, the risks and the outcomes of surgery, future monitoring and adjuvant therapy, of who else needs to be told, and at what level of detail. Medical ethics frame discourse around the risks of treatment, stipulate informed consent, and provide ways of preventing, informing and managing adverse events. In medical discourse, disclosure centres on the communication of knowledge of a person's health (or illness) status, or the potential to develop an illness in time, as suggested by the example of cancer (above) or of Huntington's disease (Flaherty, Preloran and Browner, this volume). Thus disclosure includes questions of the etiology, diagnosis and prognosis of a given condition, the propensity for illness, and its transmission and risk to others. The dilemmas of truth telling in such circumstances have increased in recent years with the growing confidence of geneticists and clinicians to understand the development of disease, the improved sensitivity of diagnostic and screening technologies, increased access to such technologies, and a growing expectation that people will wish to take advantage of these. The dilemmas of truth telling have intensified, therefore, with expectations that people already identified as at risk will undergo specific tests and act in ways concordant with the results. From this point, screening becomes routine, creating an increasing need (if unmet, in global terms) for counselling to ensure informed consent and to help people decide on action, including how to disclose their diagnosis to loved ones and others. Here, the imperative of disclosure produces specific social relations, as the discloser seeks out relations of support and service, and reflects on and acts in accordance with understandings of personal morality and ethical responsibility.

While ethical considerations shape theoretical understandings and the practical use of genetic diagnostic technology, the information produced through this technology must necessarily be disclosed to the owners of the genetic material in terms of advice on reproductive futures and the possibilities of disease in future generations (Hanssen 2004, Hertogh et al. 2004, Padilla et al. 2008, Root 2010). Flaherty, Pleloran and Browner (this volume) illustrate this in relation to Huntington's disease, when they highlight distinct local understandings of medical, biological and personal knowledge, and so draw attention to the challenges in clinical medicine and public health in relation to truth, revelation and risk.

Increasingly, disclosure is shaped by technological change, as occurs when the possibility of developing an illness and its probable trajectory can be mapped out. Individuals who are directly affected must determine who should do the telling, and make decisions about the social actions that follow from the disclosure. New forms of biomedical care intensify requirements of patient disclosure to diagnose and treat diseases and to prevent their onward transmission to progeny or in sexual life. Discourse on disclosure in these fields of action attends especially to the reasoning, processes and implications of disclosing in biomedical (or biosocial and medical) fields.

But disclosure is complicated by inequalities of power and cultural ideas of truthtelling. Joe Kaufert (1999), drawing on ethnographic work with native Canadian communities in Manitoba, and Elizabeth Bennett (1999), with the Isaan in northern Thailand, highlighted the elasticity of this simple understanding of the right to know, and the relative role of people within given social networks – families and health professionals – of managing, translating and relaying information. In the case of illness trajectories and end-of-life decisions, senior health professionals may initiate disclosure, but who receives the disclosed information varies, as does their capacity to make sense of the knowledge imparted (Bennett 1999, Kaufert 1999). Moreover, social and structural status determines the occasion, content and comprehension of specific truths. Even the apparently simple act of relaying a diagnosis can be fraught with cultural, moral and ethical challenges, including who to tell and how much information, with what spin, to provide.

A focus on clinical disclosure elides the fact that any disclosure has a social life. The disclosure is not simply given and received in a consulting room. In any intimate relationship, for instance, questions of the body and its genetic provenance become relevant. Individuals grapple with the timing of when it is appropriate to reveal that they have (for example) a colostomy, that they carry the genetic markers for breast cancer, or that they had a parent who had died of suicide or a cousin in jail for sex crimes; they rehearse their capacity to speak about and address questions of inheritance, influence and trust. People often get the moment of timing wrong, too, for there is no 'right time' to disclose some facts of the self. Hence, people often choose to withhold knowledge, where it is not culpable, to ensure privacy and to avoid intrusion, so as to manage various social interactions and perceptions. People may, for example, elect to withhold a diagnosis from others even in the case of non-communicable disease, not to disguise the risk of transmission, but to manage other people's emotional responses to diagnosis and so to contain others' inquiries into their health and how they live their lives (with respect to diabetes, see Kokanovic and Manderson 2006).

While Goffman's ideas of stigma help us understand these considerations, his work on impression management is equally relevant here (1959, 1963). The management of 'essential truths' of the person occurs in relation to various problematic health conditions, including infections, as indicated above with respect to HIV, and for leprosy and TB, but also in relation to degenerative and potentially fatal conditions (multiple sclerosis, haemophilia and Alzheimer's disease). The management of truth is perhaps especially relevant for mental health conditions, even for very common conditions such as depression (Kokanovic and Philip, this volume), and for sleep disorders (Wolf-Meyer, this volume). People in paid employment are often mindful of the potential economic costs of disclosure, but also may be mindful that public disclosure can work strategically to ward off further invasions of privacy, and dilute any fear of risk of exposure by others. I am thinking here of trans people who, by choosing the timing of their disclosure of their gender identity, pre-empt their exposure by others (Vernon, this volume).

Technologies of telling

Historical traditions of truth telling, such as the confessional in religious traditions routinely and at end of life, suggest that disclosing matters are revelatory of the individual (Hymer 1995), and that the failure to tell is morally and emotionally corrosive, so reinforcing the idea of the confession as normalising (Foucault 1978, Munro and Randall 2007). The contrived confessions and disclosures of false consciousness, that symbolically marked the end of one life (capitalism, bourgeois desire) and augured a new life (for instance, under communism), extend this notion of the power of telling. Recent examples highlight the power of the confessional to manipulate the public. For example, Tonda (2001) illustrates how prophets and anti-sorcery pastors emerged at the centre of ethnic and national conflicts in the Congo, challenging other established political, medical and religious relations. This is not unique to religious and quasi-religious practice. However, the apprehension of criminals partly depends on the willingness of people to come forward to confess a crime, as an act preferable to the lifelong surveillance of the self to avoid exposure, and interrogational techniques shaped to elicit the confession and establish remorse (Kidwell and Martinez 2010, Martel 2010).

At the same time, the increased bureaucratisation of everyday life and the rationalisation of education, work and law, to name a few, means that increasingly publics are asked to disclose facts about our lives, bodies, minds and pecuniary and material interests, at times with unintended consequences. Exposures that occur through Wikileaks, Facebook and other social media are flashpoints for strenuous debate about privacy, implying that a new politics of disclosure is taking shape in a densely networked world. Social research, too, depends on research participants' willingness to share their life stories, often on the claim that the telling will produce both personal and wider social good.

Disclosure therefore leads us to consider the dynamics of secrecy and truth telling, broadcast and exposure, in public and private domains. Ideas of the 'truth' of personhood and identity, distilled through specific 'facts' of the self, and notions of interpersonal responsibility, shape how secrecy and secrets, privacy and confidentiality are upheld, unsettled or resisted in particular settings (Bharadwaj 2003, Crook 1999, George 1993). Within families, for instance, the value of privacy, the maintenance of secrecy, the cost of confidentiality breaches, and the power that these values exercise over individuals, can have deep repercussions, as discussed in relation to abortion or fertility control, for instance, but also in relation to questions of infidelity and sexual abuse, or, in different cultural contexts, to questions of female genital cutting or male initiation, when disclosure across gender or ritual boundaries threatens social coherence (see Boddy, this volume).

Further, communication technology has reshaped how people disclose, to whom they disclose, and how they protect themselves from unintended disclosure. For example, e-health is figured, in part, around the circulation of knowledge on health status, health and bodily aspirations, and other aspects of identity, and disclosure of a particular identity marker is a prerequisite to belonging to many online as well as in-life biocommunities, even when the information disclosed, and its associated identity, cannot be verified (Davis and Flowers, this volume). Increasingly, health care too is delivered by communication technologies, with disclosure the mechanism by which to gain access to care and support. Thus medical and communication technologies have contributed to our concern with disclosure: the effects of technologies of disclosure on social relationships, wellbeing and life circumstances; the slippages that routinely occur between secrecy, confidentiality, disclosure and exposure; and the implications of these for self-presentation, social relations and sociality.

As the above illustrates, disclosures occur at multiple levels. These include the proximate context of the telling; the choice of the person who is recipient of the disclosure; the presentation of self often politically and morally; the role of the discloser to others who are part of the account of disclosure; the nature of social relationships revealed in the context of disclosing; the emotional response of the discloser to the positions that others might have adopted; and the emotionality (or its absence) in the act of story-telling. These are not 'small stories' of everyday lives, as Janet Boddy (this volume) uses the term. Rather, small stories emerge in the sequencing of stories of disclosure, with each small story containing a new revelation and account of the self. Even the simplest most economic disclosure – 'I am HIV' (Davis and Flowers, this volume) – does more than inform the listener of the discloser's viral status. The metonym reveals much of how an infection, by virtue of its history, and its significance in shaping both the present and the future, comes to dominate an ordinary life. At the same time, the economy in telling leads the discloser and disclosee to reflect on the emotional impact of HIV, and its capacity to render almost mute those living with the virus. A disclosure is not (only) the words that are voiced, but the gestures, demeanour, silences and tears that accompany different matters of disclosure in different contexts and settings. The embodiment of nervousness, anxiety, fear or relief, or the display of any other emotion, frame the act of disclosure and invite or discourage inquiry from the disclosee. These facts in turn provide openings for, or close off, the potential for further disclosures.

In the public domain

Individual and government decisions to contain and prevent disclosure have much in common as strategies to maintain social order. The possible outcome of disclosure, even in the personal instance of telling someone about HIV status, is to destabilise and disrupt; the outcome of exposure is intentionally to destabilise the individual. But any disclosure can destabilise in unanticipated ways. Researchers of war and violence routinely uncover the complicity of neighbours, relatives and friends in war; anyone might be deeply implicated in times of chaos and violence. Sometimes, one person's disclosure is another person's nightmare, since any disclosure involves, by definition, more than one person, no act of disclosure is innocent of effect.

Over many decades, people who have felt vulnerable to the risks of disclosure, or of exposure – that is, the disclosure of the personal by others – have argued the protective value of politicising the relation of the personal, private realm and the public. Coming out, for instance, was a strategic act to make the private public in order to reduce social exclusion, bullying and discrimination. When sexuality and gender identity were reasons for blackmail, it was arguably safer to be out publically than in the closet. But sexuality is only one such example: consider the risks of exposure, secrecy and fear that inform the knowledge management of personal experience (as perpetrator or victim) of torture, sexual violence, bankruptcy, fraud, imprisonment, heroin addiction or homicide. While disclosure is a nuanced act, it is at times represented in simple terms, often with the medicalisation of a given condition, state or identity that might or might not be told in a particular context – sexuality and gender identity fall into this domain. But disclosure includes acts of uncovering knowledge (and secrets) and making such knowledge public – exposing individuals and their actions, and understanding the significance and costs of silence where for political, social or personal reasons, a person, a family, or a community chooses not to disclose certain knowledge and states.

People who have fallen into any of these backgrounds are marked irrevocably. People often carefully manage their life stories, because to disclose is to revisit personal pain and emotional discomfort. By way of example, consider the strategic silences of people who have survived war, terror and oppression: the passivity and muteness of people who have survived multiple abuses including under the Pol Pot and communist regimes in Cambodia, as Sotheara Chhim (2012) describes it; or the silences of refugees in Australia and their small stories of truth spoken in spaces of absolute trust and confidence. In contrast, consider how public examples of disclosure indelibly reconstruct identities. Melbourne journalist Kate Holden (2012) is one example, who, in a memoir and a summary newspaper article, came out as a former heroin addict and sex worker. Her motivation, as she explained in an interview, is instructive: 'I think I was happy to admit frailty, fragility and vulnerability in my memoirs because they were true of me, and not shameful, and certainly once I'd published the first one I understood that my vulnerability being revealed seemed to make readers feel better about their own . . . in the second book I was prepared to make myself look very stupid and vulnerable' (Holden 2012). Most people can ill afford to reveal themselves, or be revealed, as stupid and vulnerable, or as evil, mad, dangerous or simply lacking judgement, because of the personal and economic repercussions of doing so.

To some extent, because of the manipulations of secrecy in these and related examples, we have moved from individual to public (and group) acts of disclosure, and their underlying philosophy of truth telling as healing. The South African Truth and Reconciliation Commission, and the similarly entitled commissions in Canada, Liberia and Rwanda, and other committees of inquiry where giving evidence has been seen to be healing – such as the Northern Territory (Australian) Inquiry into the Protection of Aboriginal Children from Sexual Abuse and the inquiry into British Child Migration to Australia – illustrate how people participate in public acts of disclosure. The impetus for such disclosures is twofold. Firstly, those who have done wrong are exposed and, in this, justice is effected. Secondly, those wronged gain closure: disclosure is presumed to be cathartic. But exposure and disclosure have uneven effects, and there has been some ambivalence about their value. In Cambodia and in the Solomon Islands, for example, disclosures and exposures of human rights violations have at times reopened rather than healed the wounds of ethnic tension. People may construe either silence or speech as conciliatory acts. Ideas of 'healing' as inherent in public acts of disclosure (like more private acts of disclosure, as already discussed) do not always translate comfortably across cultural domains (Wyndham and Read 2010).

Disclosure, as discussed above, is broadly defined to be revelations of the self, confessions and admissions that tell something of the essential self. For this reason, they are often also risky, revealing the speaker as vulnerable, as Holden's example indicates. Exposure is the revelation by another, as occurs, for instance, in journalist inquiry, legal processes or social history, as reflected in the exposures that occurred during the Leveson Inquiry (2012) in the UK in relation to phone tapping, or as has occurred in relation to Julian Assange around rape and Wikileaks (Den Heijer 2013). Arguably these two examples are matters of public interest, truth, political manipulation and personal style, but through exposure, they are also revelations to the public of the ways in which people might be undone and institutions destabilised, of how politics works, and about the interpenetration of the political and personal, public and private. In drawing on these examples, and their elevation to fables by which to live, we gain insights into the moral imperatives and economics of truth telling that have shaped truth practices in different country settings. These include in societies where whistle blowing, leaks and scandals occur on a regular basis as a result of ideas of the public's 'right to know' certain facts, and the fallout of such acts of exposure depending on who takes on the role of exposing. These accounts are balanced by stories that remain untold or partly told, and the politics of silence and containment that shape these circumstances. As examples, these include the containment of the truth of Chernobyl and Japan's more recent post-tsunami nuclear accident at Fukushima, where the exposure is of government rather than individuals (Petryna 2003, Funabashi and Kitazawa 2012).

Focusing critically on disclosure provides us with a mechanism to 'rethink' stigma and truth telling in productive ways. It enables us to analyse the cultural suppositions that inform truth acts in private domains, and opens the way also to question the practices of telling and showing in museums and memorials, commissions of inquiry and truth and reconciliation hearings, and via the public press and online media. Disclosure takes us beyond interpersonal and intimate relations, reproduction and sexuality, health, medical and family history, to reflect also on ownership of biomaterials and custodianship; bioethics and public morality; secrecy and lies; and the ownership of and access to bio- and personal information. Moreover, these specific ways of embodying the emotions of disclosure, and the circumstance to be disclosed, in turn are new small disclosures, reflecting the previous effects or the anticipated impact of a specific disclosure. Decisions about whether or not to disclose are therefore also influenced by presumptions about the impact of disclosing, based on prior experience and witness of the effects of disclosure on others' lives. Stories are attached to any disclosure, and the unpredictability of response is a telling indicator of what is at risk. The person must therefore weigh up contradictory possible outcomes of rejection and acceptance, recrimination and vindication, to frame decisions about disclosing. What is disclosed, and to whom, is never a singular act; others are always involved because of their relationship to the discloser, historically and in the present, and have some ownership on the facts that are disclosed.

Disclosing therefore has a powerful impact for the discloser and disclosee well beyond the moment of telling. And, in telling, the discloser relinquishes their control of their story in a number of ways. Take, for instance, public disclosure in the context of a commission of inquiry, which provides a formal mechanism to tell and to be heard. The rhetoric around disclosure implies that, in recount and witness, the speaker will find closure. But it is improbable that the discloser will ever walk away with the past neatly packaged, or that he or she will no longer revisit and be haunted by the particular truth that he or she has shared. Furthermore, the particular truths cease to have a life of their own, no longer the property of the discloser but a prototype or exemplar of the experiences that shape the public inquiry and invite further inquiry, disclosure, revision and meaning making.

Concluding remarks

Disclosure is routinely characterised as a moral act, whether enacted in a public or a private domain, and regardless of the purposes of telling. Dominant and normative understandings and values shape acts of disclosure, inquiry and exposure, although these vary in time and place. In different cultural, political and institutional contexts, at quite different levels, narrative, speech acts, lexicon, discourse and silence are crafted and interpreted. Certainty and confusion are contained, managed and/or produced in everyday speech, in formal and rhetorical exchanges, in texts of different kinds, and through performance. The chapters that follow pick up these points and, in doing so, highlight the value of close interrogation of actions that we gloss as disclosures.

There has been surprisingly little critical attention of how and what people disclose, question and expose, for what purposes, and in what ways. As I have already suggested, questions of disclosure, exposure and concealment have extended widely to include ethical positions and epistemological challenges in relation to politics, citizenship, sociality and government. In this volume we begin the task of a nuanced and systematic account of disclosure and what this implies for the constitution of human subjectivity and social relations. In distinctive and yet intersecting ways, we are engaged with matters that might be confidential, deeply private and rarely voiced, and we are engaged with the management, revelation, control and dissemination of such knowledge. We have not explored, to the depth that is warranted, the affective dimensions of disclosure, although this is surely paramount in establishing the salience of particular disclosures and in elucidating what is at stake in so doing. Yet disclosure perhaps always has emotional valency and convolution, with the content, timing and manner of disclosure all revealing much of the self, identity and relationality.

In the chapters that follow, authors from anthropology, sociology and psychology have drawn on their analytic approaches to disclosure, with a mutual interest in the enactment of disclosure. They examine ways of telling stories that often render the storyteller vulnerable. More than a linking thematic for this volume, the idea of disclosure raises important questions that affect people in everyday life, recurrently and recursively. It frames our contemporary research practices and our relationships with the people we study. It raises questions of the tensions that emerge between private and public good, and it forces us to think about silence and knowledge, the imperative to tell, the right to know, and the right to privacy.

2 Stories told in passing?

Disclosure in narratives of everyday lives in Andhra Pradesh

Janet Boddy

> Narratives are keyed both to the events in which they are told and to the events that they recount.
>
> Bauman 1986: 2

In this chapter, I reflect on the performative nature of disclosure in families' accounts of their everyday lives and practices, questioning the meanings of disclosure within the identity performance of stories told in interviews.

The term 'disclosure' has many meanings. *The Oxford English Dictionary* (OED Online 2013) refers to 'the action of disclosing or opening up to view; revelation; discovery, exposure'. The implication here is of bringing to light something previously hidden, an understanding of disclosure that is familiar in social research with children and families. The research ethics literature similarly highlights 'disclosure' in relation to participants' revelation of information that would otherwise be concealed, or is a cause for concern. For example, the UK's major social science research funding body, the Economic and Social Research Council (ESRC), has a Framework for Research Ethics (2010: 9–10) which specifically highlights potential for disclosure as a risk factor in research, 'in particular, where participants are persuaded to reveal information which they would not otherwise disclose in the course of everyday life . . . [or] where the research topic or data gathering involves a risk of information being disclosed that would require the researchers to breach confidentiality conditions agreed with participants'.

Is it possible to go beyond this risk-focused conceptualisation of disclosure? Other chapters in this volume question the conceptualisation of disclosure as problematic, for example, in relation to major life disruptions (e.g. Flaherty, Preloran and Browner, this volume). Lenore Manderson, in this volume, discusses disclosure as a social act, highlighting the need to recognise the function of any disclosure within its social context: not only what is told, but to whom and for what reason. If the research interview is understood as a site of identity performance, the act of telling – of disclosure – can be seen as part of the participant's identity construction, allowing the researcher to move beyond an assumption of risk, shame or stigma.

The analysis which I present in this chapter aims to add to the shades of disclosure detailed through this volume, examining the appearance of the apparently secret or difficult to tell amidst the more prosaic sharing of stories of everyday life. By considering the research interview as a form of conversation, and focusing on the work that is done by the 'small stories' of everyday lives – with all their inconsistencies and equivocations – it is possible to recognise disclosure as part of the co-constructed nature of telling, and so not confined to revelations of significant or adverse events. It is also important to consider tellability in what is or is not said. Are the small stories told in interviews really told 'in passing'? Or are disclosures co-constructed, within narratives framed for (and by) the interviewer in the context of that interview, and his or her research focus and questioning?

The research

The analysis presented here draws on data from an ongoing study of family lives and the environment. The research is part of a UK ESRC National Centre for Research Methods (NCRM) Node, NOVELLA,[1] which comprises several projects that apply narrative approaches to the study of everyday family lives. Here, I reflect on work conducted for the first phase of the Family Lives and Environment study: a narrative secondary analysis of research interviews conducted with families in Andhra Pradesh (India).

The overall aim of the Family Lives and Environment study is to improve understanding of the negotiated complexity of families' lives in relationship with their environments, with regard to meanings of 'environment' in everyday family lives and family practices. Elizabeth Shove (2010) has written critically about over-simplification in relation to climate change research. Approaches to the development of (environmentally) sustainable practices are often rooted in attitude and behaviour change, and in economic models, both of which neglect social theory. She has commented that 'climate change policy proceeds on the basis of an extraordinarily limited understanding of the social world and is, for the most part, untouched by theoretical debate of any kind' (Shove 2010: 278). Similarly, Ramsay and Manderson (2011: 180) wrote of the need for climate change policy to address the complexity of subjective experience among individuals, families and communities 'to explore more deeply the relationship between the human spirit and the physical world'. How can deeper understandings be achieved?

The study seeks to exemplify the variety of families' lived experiences in contrasting contexts within and between countries, through case studies of family life in India and the UK. The project's focus on India and the UK is designed to trouble questions of translatability in cross-national research and to illuminate the potential for shared learning between countries with very different economic, social, cultural and demographic profiles. Hulme (2009) wrote that 'developing' countries are frequently portrayed as needing the help of the developed world to respond to climate change. But what are the lessons for economically affluent nations from the experience of those living in lower income countries?

The demarcation between 'developed' and 'developing' nations is not straightforward. Whilst rapid economic growth and urbanisation in India has prompted concern about the growth of consumption among affluent sub-groups within the population (Myers and Kent 2003; Revi 2008), the vast majority of the Indian population has not experienced affluent consumerism (Galab et al. 2008). Global North paradigms of sustainability and lower consumption may be of questionable relevance to nations such as India where climatic events such as droughts or floods disproportionately affect the lives of certain groups in the population, notably the rural poor (e.g. Morrow and Vennam 2009).

Against this context, the Family Lives and Environment study began with a case-based narrative secondary analysis of interviews from eight family case studies conducted in Andhra Pradesh, a state of 85 million people in south-eastern India, as part of Young Lives, an ongoing international longitudinal cohort study of childhood poverty, involving approximately 12,000 families in four countries (Ethiopia, India, Peru and Vietnam). Core funded by the UK Department for International Development (DFID), Young Lives started in 2001–2 as a child-focused household survey; a qualitative component was added in 2006; the study runs until 2017. To date, three rounds of qualitative data have been collected, and a fourth is being developed at the time of writing. The qualitative longitudinal research is designed to complement and extend the quantitative cohort study, using a multi-method approach to examine how poverty interacts with other factors at individual, household, community and inter-generational levels to shape children's life trajectories over time. The Young Lives qualitative longitudinal research (QLR), according to the researchers, aims 'to capture both what we as researchers assume to be relevant and important (e.g. the move from one school to a different school, or death of a parent) and what our research participants view as important (e.g. a child describing as a "turning point" the day when he was given his own small plot of land to cultivate on the family farm)' (Crivello, Morrow and Streuli 2013: 2). The QLR involves 200 children (and their caregivers) across the four study countries – 48 families in Andhra Pradesh – and includes an older cohort (aged 12–13 years at the time of the first interview) and a younger cohort (aged 6–7 years at the time of the first interview).[2]

The eight cases re-analysed for Family Lives and Environment comprise a tiny fraction of the families involved in the main Young Lives study, and even in the qualitative sub-sample. They were drawn from the older cohort sample in Andhra Pradesh, and were purposely sampled in relation to the substantive objectives of the Family Lives and Environment study. They were not intended to be representative of Young Lives families, either in India or more generally, but were sampled as cases with the potential to inform our understanding of family practices and everyday lives as they relate to the environment (broadly defined to range from everyday local environments – sites for everyday family practices – to major events and concerns, including environmental shocks such as drought). The eight cases included four boys and four girls, living in families in rural and urban contexts.

For each of the eight family cases, six transcripts were analysed in depth – interviews with caregivers and children over three rounds of data collection. This was supplemented with contextual reading of group interviews with children, and interviews with community leaders. This secondary analysis examined ways in which experiences and understandings of environment (and environmental concerns) were woven into narratives within family members' accounts of their lives. An additional aim was to inform methodological development for a later stage of fieldwork with a new sample of families in India and the UK.

In this chapter, I focus on just one case – Rahmatullah (pseudonym)[3] and his family – an Urdu-speaking Muslim family living in a city of several million people. The family were first interviewed when Rahmatullah was 11 years old; the second interview took place one year later and the third was just over three years after the initial interview, when he was 15 years old. At the time of the third interview, the family had experienced major disruption in their lives with the death of Rahmatullah's older brother, the primary wage earner. I have selected this case because of its potential to illustrate the intersection between the young person's experiences and responsibilities within the family, and his relationship with his lived environment, over time and in the context of the emotional and practical consequences of this significant bereavement.

Narratives in context

There are obvious limits on the contextual understanding that frames a secondary analysis such as that reported here, conducted at significant temporal and geographic distance from the context of the original interview and at a substantive distance from the original objectives of the study. For the purposes of this chapter, I have focused on Rahmatullah and his family because their interviews can illuminate the performative nature of 'disclosure' in narratives of everyday life. However, Langellier (1999: 128) comments that 'approaching personal narrative as performance requires theory which takes context as seriously as it does text'. Her observation highlights an important caveat for the analysis reported here, which entailed very close reading of a single case – akin to the close-up of a macro-zoom camera lens, in comparison to the wide-angle reading of a cross-case analysis (as intended in the Young Lives QLR research). The risk is that one may see the trees, but not the forest.

My secondary analysis also crossed countries and languages, and this has particular implications for narrative analysis in several respects. There are questions about understanding the cultural and contextual nature of genre story forms, given the difference between my cultural formation (UK born, of European origin) and that of the Young Lives interview team in Andhra Pradesh. In addition, interviews for Young Lives in Andhra Pradesh were conducted in local languages – Rahmatullah's family were interviewed in Urdu – and recorded, transcribed and translated into English. Narrative analysis usually focuses closely on the particular linguistic devices used in story telling (e.g. Bauman 1986, Riessman 2003), but close reading and line-by-line analysis – attending to choice of words, or examining repetitions, for example – may not be warranted when interviews are read in translation, and were not transcribed with narrative analytic reading in mind. As Fox (2008: 342) observes, 'there is no possibility of literal translation having the same meaning in both languages'.

Given these challenges, the framework in which the research was conducted is important. The overarching aim of the National Centre for Research Methods – the centre within which my project is based – is to foster methodological innovation. One key methodological objective for the Family Lives and Environment project was, in effect, to consider what is possible – what (or whether) a narrative analysis can contribute. Addressing these challenges has critically depended on attention to context, enabled through close collaboration and discussion not only with the core Family Lives and Environment researchers, but equally with the Young Lives qualitative research teams in the UK and in India (see Acknowledgements) – for example, through access to data gathering reports which contextualise the interview data, and through questioning and discussing readings of the data. The analysis presented here is my own, but it has been informed by discussion with this wider team.

Disclosing everyday life

To understand the relationship between family lives and understandings and experiences of environment, it is necessary to attend to the materiality of everyday life (Miller 2012). Shove writes that 'stuff comes to matter in social theory' (2010: 280). Halkier and colleagues (2011: 6) talked about 'the material environment . . . central in the process of creating interaction, continuity and reality'. Materiality is also central to theories of practice, and to theorising practices in relation to consumption, drawing on theorists such as Reckwitz (2002), Schatzki (2001) and Warde (2005). As Warde (2005: 137) wrote, 'consumption is not in itself a practice but is, rather, a moment in almost every practice'.

The focus of Family Lives and Environment is on what Halkier and colleagues (2011: 6) term 'the practice of everyday life', and its relationship with the 'quotidian spaces' in which families live (Moran 2005). In this focus, the study forms part of a growing body of work concerned with understanding – and telling – the everyday. Scott (2009) notes that the study of everyday life can sometimes be assumed to be trivial or mundane. Indeed, the very nature of the everyday – trivial or mundane, and easily forgotten – makes it difficult to research (Boddy and Smith 2008). Is everyday life, then, hidden from (the researcher's) view – and difficult to disclose?

Hitchings (2011) noted that researchers studying everyday life appear increasingly hesitant about using interview methods to study routine practices, given the disconnections between what people do and what they say they do. Ethnographic and particularly observational approaches are often seen as better suited to studying the everyday, precisely because everyday life is not readily disclosable. Miller (2012), for example, argues convincingly for the importance of long-term ethnographic fieldwork as an essential method for understanding consumption in everyday life, and Pink's (2009: 19) 'sensory ethnography' is designed to capture 'the multisensoriality of how people experience their homes, material cultures and domestic products and practices'. However, Hitchings (2011) argues that interviews are worthwhile in studying everyday lives and practices, because of what we do when we *tell* of our everyday lives – when we disclose or reveal our lives. Interviews can provide a way of examining the meanings that are made of everyday life, and the ways in which practices can be framed (for example in relation to identities).

To understand everyday lives in families, we also need to recognise that we are not simply individual practitioners. We must attend to 'the sets of relationships (structures, collectivities) within which these activities are carried out and from which they derive their meaning' (Morgan 2011, no page numbers). Practices are embedded in social worlds. Abstract theories of practice have been criticised (e.g. Warde 2005) for being insufficiently attentive to the social processes involved, and for neglecting agency and decision making, for over-emphasising Reckwitz's (2002) idea that as practitioners we are captured by our practices. Hargreaves (2011: 83) wrote that 'social practice theory thus diverts attention away from moments of individual decision making', and Hitchings (2011: 62) criticised the conceptualisation of 'people as the unwitting "carriers" of practices by which they have previously been infected'.

This work implies a need to attend to agency, to recognise that we are not merely carriers of practice. Equally, there is a need to recognise that we do not only function as individuals; practices, and decisions about practices, are relational, dynamic, negotiated and maintained within wider social structures and within everyday family lives. Narrative analysis, with its focus on meaning-making, provides a valuable way into understanding the disclosure of family practices and their relationship to individual and collective identities within families.

Given that practices are connected, not only socially but within time and space, and given the emphasis of narrative analysis on progression and connections across symbols and themes (see Squire 2008), a narrative approach should be particularly useful in illuminating the social, spatial and temporal nature of family practices. At the same time, the research on which I draw aims to illuminate the ways in which habitual practices – and materiality within those practices – fit into the 'told story' of the interview narrative.

Disclosure and narrative analysis

Manderson (this volume) illuminates the nature of disclosure as a social act. A key feature of narration is its performative and communicative nature: stories are told in interaction (Riessman 2003). Phoenix (2008) writes that analysis of the 'small story' – brief and topically descriptive – enables attention to the performative work done by narratives in interview interactions. Small stories are thus especially relevant to understanding disclosure as a social act within an interview. They can also provide insights into 'canonical narratives' (Bruner 1991) – reflecting participants' understandings of (and response to) socially and culturally accepted norms. For example, in Riessman's (2000) study of south Indian childless women, women's agency was highlighted by 'disclosures' of resistance to hegemonic norms within small stories of everyday life.

To understand the role of disclosure in narrative, it is important to consider Bruner's (1991) observation that both the storyteller and the listener must consider the background knowledge of the other. Disclosures are made within the context of this perceived knowledge, based not only on what is *asked* in an interview, but on a judgement of what needs to be told or explained or justified. This conceptualisation of disclosure – of what is told or revealed in the interview context – can include that which is neatly storied, but can also attend to that which is not readily disclosed, which is absent, or incoherent, or which does not 'fit' with the dominant narrative in the interview (Phoenix 2008).

Phoenix's observations about narrative coherence resonate with Hermans' (e.g. 2003) discussion of the complex and narratively structured dialogic self, characterised by discontinuities between different 'I' voices. Hermans argues that the self has multiple potentially contradictory stories and, in this context, disclosure can be seen as a way of managing presentation of the dialogic self – the stories that are told bring to light particular 'I' voices. This is not about disclosure of objective 'truth', nor is it restricted to disclosures of risk or of harm. Rather, by recognising disclosure as a social act of revelation, in the context of the performative nature of the interview interaction, we can gain insight into the meanings that are made of everyday lives and the ways in which individual and family identities may be constructed in accounts of everyday lives. As Riessman (2003: 337) observes, 'informants negotiate how they want to be known by the stories they develop collaboratively with their audiences'. Through disclosure, the participant can endeavour to manage the aspects of their selves and lives that are revealed within the context of the research encounter.

Rahmatullah and his family

Is the conceptualisation of disclosure outlined above – as part of a performative narrative of individual and family identity – relevant to understanding the everyday lives of Rahmatullah and his family, as told in the interviews they gave within the Young Lives study? As detailed above, the Young Lives qualitative subsample provides a longitudinal data set with multiple perspectives including young people and caregivers. This means that narratives may emerge or be discernible within cases (across time and/or data sources), within single interviewees' accounts across time, or within single interviews.

Rahmatullah

Rahmatullah and his family participated in Round 1 interviews when he was only 11 years old, living with his mother, father and siblings in a large city in the state of Andhra Pradesh. At the beginning of his first interview, Rahmatullah appears to set out an identity position which he develops over the course of the interview – and, in fact, over all three rounds of data collection – as a responsible member of the family, informed and involved. This can be seen from the beginning of the first interview, when the interviewer seeks to ensure that Rahmatullah understands the aims and nature of the study for the purposes of ensuring informed consent.

I: Did you ask your mother why this aunty [the researcher] has come? And what I will ask?
R: She said that yesterday you came and today you will come by 10 o'clock. I told fine, and went to get the provisions. And today I asked again that it's already 10 and they did not come. She said they might have not come. And I watched the cycle shop where the vehicles are parked. . . . Saw that all of you were leaving in the vehicle yesterday. And today I saw while you were coming.

This small story of watching and waiting could be seen to begin to establish a canonical narrative of the good son, conscientious, observant and helpful. This identity position is elaborated through a variety of 'small stories' across the three rounds of data collection, as Rahmatullah discloses details of his everyday practices. Such disclosures undoubtedly reflect the interviewer's questioning – about his daily life and time use – but they also serve to evidence and reinforce his narrative. He tells stories of everyday life at school, and later at work, that illustrate his support for and involvement with everyday family life and his growing responsibilities in the family. Rahmatullah's account accords with Vennam's and Komanduri's (2009: 18) analysis of Young Lives Round 1 interviews in India, which highlights gendered experiences of growing responsibility for boys and girls in the sample: boys are 'considered to be more responsible and are expected to move and carry out work independently'. As for other children in the Young Lives India sample, for Rahmatullah the growth of responsibility and of spatial mobility were inseparable. This is evident across interviews in his accounts of growing up. For example, in Round 1 the interviewer asks him how he has changed in the last year:

I: When you were in sixth class, what were you like?
R: I was good.
I: Ah, you were good then also. Do you feel you have grown taller like that?
R: Yes, grown taller.
I: What else?
R: Grown taller, and able to understand better. I know to get things and became familiar with routes to far off places. I can understand better. Even if there is a quarrel in front of us, I know how to resolve it.

Spatial mobility, linked to his growing expertise and responsibility, emerges again in small stories told in the Round 2 interview. For example, the interviewer asks Rahmatullah what has changed since her last visit. He replies:

R: Now, I am clever in getting provisions, now I go to *mandi* [a bigger market, further away] and get the groceries.
I: Last year you did not go there?
R: No.
I: Why?
R: My father used to go, now he is not going, his health is not good.
I: Why do you go, why can't your elder brothers go?
R: They go for work . . . As there is no one at home, I will go for it.

In Round 3, when Rahmatullah is 15 years old, the interviewer again asks how his life has changed.

I: If Rahmatullah turns back and looks in the past at these 15 years, what was he doing?
R: Go to school, come, bring groceries, work, go for tuition, and if I find time, go out and play.
I: He used to do all those things, now what is Rahmatullah doing?
R: Get up in the morning, bring milk packet, eat food, go to the shop [where R now works]. Come back in the evening and bring tablets . . .
I: In all these works, which work did you like the most?
R: The work I used to do before?
I: Yes.
R: Going and getting groceries and doing this and that.

Rahmatullah's account of his everyday life shows his practices as collectively negotiated within and for the family. His small stories of daily life are consistent with wider themes in the Young Lives qualitative analysis (e.g. Vennam and Komandura 2009), but in narrative terms they also accord with a wider normative (or canonical) narrative of his responsibility and commitment to the family.

Buitelaar (2006: 262) writes that the formation of identity is a process of orchestrating voices within the self that speak from different I-positions, as a basis for self-disclosure that depends on 'the actual or imagined positions from which self-narrations are told'. The examples given above relate to an identity position that Rahmatullah foregrounds for the interviewer, beginning with the small story with which he responds to the interviewer's first question. He is a responsible young man, committed to his family. To highlight this positioning is not to question (or even to evaluate) its truth, but rather simply to note the consistency of the (co)construction of this identity position throughout the interviews. His narratives of daily life highlight two key features of his life, as he tells it. First, in his detailed lists, as in the example quoted in Round 3, he both emphasises and evidences how much he does for his family: 'Get up in the morning, bring milk packet, eat food, go to the shop. Come back in the evening and bring tablets.' Second, his strong 'I' voice is centred in the small stories he tells (as in the examples given here), highlighting his agency, his commitment and his expertise: 'And today I asked . . . And I watched . . . And today I saw . . . I am good . . . able to understand better . . . Now I am clever . . . now I go . . . I will go for it.'

Over the course of the interviews, while probing to capture the details of Rahmatullah's time use and daily activities (a key focus of the Young Lives qualitative research), the interviewer prompts him to talk about an aspect of his daily life which he appears hesitant to discuss at length – his engagement with play and leisure activities. By the time of the Round 3 interview – and perhaps unsurprisingly, given that he is now working full-time to support his family – Rahmatullah makes a reference to play as a limited feature of his past, but not his present life. Elsewhere in that interview, when asked what makes him happy, he says 'mostly playing', but across the three rounds of data collection, he appears to resist the interviewer's questions about play. Play – and pleasure in play – appears difficult to disclose in the context of the identity position that he foregrounds in the interviews. Certainly, there is some ambiguity and contradiction in his accounts. For example, in Round 1, when he is 11 years old, the interviewer asks him directly about play:

I: Daily for how much time you play? What do you play?
R: I . . . play for half an hour. Hide and seek, marbles, catching through holding each other's hands.
I: Like lock and key [a game]! What do you call it?
R: Chain and box.

I: Do you like kite flying?

R: Yes.

I: Have you taken any new ones [toys or games]?

R: No. I have taken that box [pointing to a Rubik's Cube] . . . All the same colours should be matched.

I: Have you tried it?

R: Yes. I did it once, but could not do it again. . . . On one side, red colour and the other side, yellow, and white

I: It's very difficult. If you can get it on one side it's great.

R: Yes.

I: What will you do in the evening?

R: By five or five thirty have to get the provisions.

I: You have to get it every day?

R: Yes. Like meat, oil, green chillies, like that . . .

I: By what time you will go?

R: By quarter past or half past five.

I: Do you play after that?

R: If I have time I will play, otherwise I get involved in the work.

I: Do your friends call you?

R: Yes they do, but I won't go. At home they tell there is work, and will allow if I have spare time.

I: Do you get angry?

R: No. I will do the work and then go to play. I will play at least once in a day.

Later in the same interview, the subject of play re-emerges, and the interviewer asks a leading question, encouraging Rahmatullah to breach the dominant narrative of the agentic responsible hard-working son:

I: These are things which you like, now you are growing, are there any things which you do not like? I will give an example like doing work always. You have told so many things but forgot to tell one thing? Think about it?

R: Feeling disgusted of always doing the work.

The interviewer's choice of example, 'like doing work always', appears to prompt a disclosure – of disgust – but Rahmatullah quickly moves away from this position in response to her further questions:

I: Are you happy of not playing much?

R: Yes. Because we will be happy while playing after that we have suffer with pains. Then we have to go to hospital and take medicines. So why [go to] all that trouble? That's why we should not play much. We should play limitedly.

I: Do you think that there will be pains if we play?

R: Yes if run for long time, jump then will have pains.

I: So do you feel it is better to stop playing?

R: We should not play for longer hours, it will be better if we grow and can go to far off places by walking.

His cautionary story of hospital and pain as a consequence of too much play appears as a morality tale, reinforced through the normative statements (e.g. 'we should not play much'). The interviewer's continued prompting in relation to his views and experiences of play is certainly consistent with the Young Lives Round 1 objective of gaining a full account of children's daily life and time use. But as a secondary analyst – even working in collaboration with the Young Lives team who conducted the interviews – there is a limit to how much I can know about the context in which his account is given, including his expression or tone of voice as he spoke (for example, whether he sounded disgusted, or if he was joking). When analysing at a distance – from a translated transcript – some things remain unknown. Nonetheless, there is an apparent ambivalence. Rahmatullah partially resists the interviewer's attempts to frame the lack of play as problematic – 'Do you get angry?' 'No. I will do the work'. But his feelings about play are further revealed later in the Round 1 interview when he is asked to remember 'one happy moment':

I: When you look back do you remember one happy moment?

R: Ah. Yes I used to play a lot in the childhood. Now, not much time to play. Earlier, used to play marbles and fly kites with friends. Now I do not do that.

This nostalgic account is placed firmly in the past through Rahmatullah's use of language: 'Now not much time . . .'; 'Earlier, used to . . . Now I do not . . .'.

This is a disclosure, but the revelation of something otherwise concealed is only glimpsed, through his momentary expression of disgust at his family responsibilities, and his nostalgia for play in earlier childhood. Neither example fits a risk-oriented definition of disclosure, of the sort discussed earlier. However, both are revelations, in offering an 'opening up to view' of a different perspective on his everyday life, a perspective that Rahmatullah has to work to situate, to minimise and distance from the I-position that is foregrounded in the interview. This distancing may be culturally normative: the Western ethic of the 'child' and the 'innocence' of play may have little relevance for non-elite Indian childhoods (Balagopalan 2011). Regardless, Rahmatullah's account illustrates the need to recognise the co-constructed nature of disclosure. His stories are not told in passing; they are prompted by the demands of the interview. But they also reveal his agency – not only in his identity as a responsible and committed son in his everyday family life, but also as a research participant, visibly managing disclosures to support his identity position in the interview.

Rahmatullah's mother

Interviews with Rahmatullah's mother indicated what might be termed an 'our-position', a collective identity framing of the family, resonating with Gillis's (1996) concept of 'the family we live by'. As with Rahmatullah's interviews, his mother's Round 1 interview develops this identity position through small stories that contribute to an over-arching narrative framing of her account of family as strong, respectable, and emotionally and economically self-sufficient, and of herself as a strong figure within the family. There are echoes throughout her account of McAdam's (1993) concept of the 'heroic narrative', highlighting achievement in the face of hardship or adversity. Rahmatullah's mother presents her family as different from others in the neighbourhood, and she tells of the ways in which the family members contribute, economically and by supporting each other. She also talks of how they are unsupported by others around them in times of adversity. Economic and material developments, such as improvements to the house, and wedding planning, elaborate the narrative of family strength that she develops over the course of the interviews, as illustrated in the following extract from the Round 2 interview:

I: The house looks new.
M: Yes, we constructed now. Earlier it was at a low level. Now we have increased the height. It was not like this at that time.

[There follows an exchange about improvements to the house.]

I: How did you manage [to pay for these changes]?
M: We put up chits [savings in instalments] and raised them. But we did not borrow from anyone.
I: How many chits did you put up or started?
M: We started three chits and raised all the three.

Rahmatullah's mother highlights the interdependence of the family, their responsibility and hard work, and the economic contributions that they each make. She also presents for herself a strong and central role, as the mother but also in carrying out and coordinating embroidery work which is done by herself and two of her children (son and daughter). Within this dominant narrative framework of the strong mother and the strong family, the father is talked about relatively little. Even when present in the room he is only mentioned briefly. In the Round 1 interview, Rahmatullah's mother first mentions her husband only in passing, as part of her response to a question about one of her sons. Later, she adds a little more information:

M: He has a hearing problem [points at father]. Because of the machines noise, he lost one ear and can't listen.
I: What was he doing?
M: Carpenter.
I: Carpenter? When did he leave that job?
M: Six years. He has problems.
I: So stays at home? Fine. Does [child] work at home? You told me about that work [embroidery work] – does he do it every day?

By the time of the Round 2 interview, the father has experienced further major health problems. Rahmatullah's mother talks about his illness in the interview, but its impact on the family is not emphasised:

I: OK, tell me about any incidents in children's life or at home circumstances?
M: The children are fine, but he [husband] was sick, we were tense. He was sick at the time of Ramadan.
I: What happened?
M: Maybe because of climate and chillness. He was unable to walk and even talk also. Even now he cannot speak out. He can tell only his name. Other than he cannot speak out anything.

[The account continues with question and answer about timing and symptoms and treatment.]

I: How much does the treatment cost there?
M: Daily it cost 200 rupees, now since few days it's costing less. Since past 2–3 months it cost 250 rupees per day. Now since 15 days it's costing less. Ever since 70–80 days it has cost this much.
I: So it has cost you much more, how have you managed?
M: I am doing it. Children also do some work and we are just managing.
I: Did you have to take loan from outside?
M: No, myself and children are managing.
I: What else happened?
M: No nothing. Everything and everybody else are fine, except him.

Although Rahmatullah's mother provides a detailed account of her family's daily life and time use, she mentions her husband little in the rest of this Round 2 interview. She makes passing reference to the fact that he does not like Rahmatullah going out, and, at the end, in response to a checking question by the interviewer, she reiterates that the father is not working because he is sick:

M: He used to do work earlier but now he is feeling cold, he is sick so I keep doing. He sits inside and keeps watching. Earlier he was doing all that, but now he is not.

I: Earlier he was doing carpenter job, is it so?

M: Yes earlier he was doing [that].

Rahmatullah's mother's framing of her husband's economic inactivity and disabling illnesses appears to minimise the impact of these events on the family, through refrains that reference the strength and self-sufficiency of the family, and her own agency in particular. This contrasts with her Round 3 interview, conducted a year after her elder son died following an unexpected illness. She introduces this news right at the beginning of the Round 3 interview:

I: How did the two years go? What all has happened?

M: After you last visited we arranged marriage for our son and had an engagement party. We celebrated the event on a grand scale. Then during Ramadan time we went to [religious site]. Two months after that he passed away. It has been one year since he passed away.

It is quite possible that the interviewer was aware of this significant event even before the formal interview started. This son was the main wage earner, and Rahmatullah's mother describes him as 'the main person' in the family. Her interview offers a powerful narrative of grief, with small self-contained narratives that tell of his death and serve to highlight the impact on the family. The loss is not simply disclosed, it is told and re-told. For example:

This house was built and everything was going on alright. The first time you came there was no house, and the second time you came this house was built and now the main person himself passed away. This is what happened in the past two years.

And later in the interview:

It affected [us] tremendously. This girl has become like this. The other son lost a lot of weight and become very skinny. The family has shattered.

But throughout the interview, Rahmatullah's mother also appears to offer a narrative of restoration (see Squire 2005 after Bruner 1990), showing how family members are retrieving 'the family they live by' in the face of their devastating loss. Through a series of small stories, she works to restore the canonical narrative of the strong and self-sufficient family that she has presented throughout the previous rounds of data collection. For example:

I: The embroidery work you are doing now, you have been doing this before your son's death too? Or did you take it up now?

M: Before we used to do this once in a while, but now we are doing it continuously and taking in more work too.

I: Does your daughter help you in embroidery work?

M: Yes. All three of us do it.

I: From where do you get this work? Do neighbourhood people give the work or do you get it from outside [the local area]?

M: We get it from outside.

I: They come to your house to give the work?

M: No we go far and bring it.

In her account, Rahmatullah's mother emphasises the family's agency – 'we are doing it', 'all three of us', 'we go far' – and in this way, she serves to highlight their cohesiveness and determination. But there is an apparent disruption in this cohesive narrative during the Round 3 interview, when she introduces new information about her husband. In previous interviews, as noted above, he plays a minimal role in her account of family life, both in the over-arching family narrative and the small stories of previous interviews. The Round 3 caregiver interview has a different dynamic because it involves Rahmatullah's mother and her mother-in-law and sister-in-law, who have returned to live with the family following their bereavement. In this interview, Rahmatullah's mother spontaneously introduces the father as a more problematic figure within the family, in an unprompted story of the events of the previous evening:

I: Did you feel that Rahmatullah has grown up and is taking responsibilities of the family?

M: Yes. He was very worried. He was worried how we are going to make ends meet. Last night his father was fighting with me for money and trying to beat me. Rahmatullah said 'don't fight, I will give you 10 rupees every day. If you both fight like this what's going to happen to us?' He took out money from his pocket and gave it to him.

I: He [the father] turned like this now or he is like this before also?

M: He is like this from the beginning. If anyone doesn't do what he wants them to do, he beats. What to do? He is like that. He says whatever he says is right.

Sister-in-law: Even if he is wrong, he still insists that he is right and every one must do what he wants. Everyone has to obey him.

I: So now Rahmatullah has started to speak out.

M: Yes.

Rahmatullah's mother says that the problem of her husband's violence is not new – 'he is like this from the beginning' – but this appears to be a new disclosure, appearing three years into the family's participation in this longitudinal study. Of course, a transcript is only a partial record of an interview encounter, and the violence may have been discussed in an unrecorded conversation with the interviewer at some point over the three rounds of data collection. But the interviewer's reaction – 'He [the father] turned like this now or he is like this before also?' – implies this is new information, previously untold. It is also more readily recognisable as a disclosure within the risk-focused definition of the term most current in Western social research, even though intimate partner violence is common in south-east Asia (including in India) in comparison to Western nations (WHO 2013).

The disclosure of her husband's violence is also unprompted (at least initially) by the interviewer, raising the question of why Rahmatullah's mother has chosen to make this revelation now. The characterisation of her husband presented here could disrupt, or contradict, the family identity that has been constructed in her previous interviews. The character of the violent husband might be seen – especially through a Western lens – to disrupt the narrative of a strong, respectable, self-sufficient family, a narrative which at times is framed in contrast to those of quarrelsome neighbours. Her previous characterisation of her husband – in poor health and reliant on the strength of the other family members – sits much more comfortably in that narrative.

This new disclosure could emerge now because trust has developed over the three years of the research relationship – perhaps, by Round 3, Rahmatullah's mother feels comfortable to disclose to the interviewer something that she previously concealed. Equally, the presence of her relatives – who support her account – could give her confidence to speak. Another reason for this disclosure might be that the family identity has already been disrupted – 'shattered' in her words – by the elder son's death. Characters may shift as the narrative is reconfigured. As noted earlier, the third interview features a recurrent narrative of restoration, in the stories the mother tells of the family's strength in coping with the eldest son's death. When reading the extract above as a complete 'small story', in Riessman's (2003) terms, we can see this as an example of restoration of the family's strength. Rahmatullah's mother's earlier reference to the eldest son's role as 'the main person' seems revealing here. Perhaps it is possible for her to problematise the father as a character because he is not such a central figure in the close-knit family canon. Over the three rounds of data collection, he is not positioned centrally in her narratives of family, whether economically or in relationships with other family members. When he is disclosed as problematic here, it happens in two ways.

First, the small story she tells here, of the incident of the previous evening, is not primarily a story about her husband. Rather, it is a story about Rahmatullah, and his responsibility and commitment to the family. This is consistent with his mother's account of him as a responsible and committed son across all three rounds of interviews although, in keeping with her characterisation of herself as a strong mother, Rahmatullah is not portrayed as perfect or idealised; he is still positioned as her child, in need of guidance and boundaries. In the Round 3 interview, this characterisation of Rahmatullah also appears to have shifted. Following his brother's death, Rahmatullah left school and started full-time work. His mother and other relatives emphasise that this was his decision, and throughout the interview they repeatedly highlight his agency and support for the family:

I: Who decided that he has to start working?
M: He himself went with a friend and got the work.
Mother-in-law: Neither father nor any brother took him and fixed in a job.
Sister-in-law: He himself searched for it and joined.

So the small story that Rahmatullah's mother tells of the previous evening could be read as developing the characterisation of Rahmatullah's agency and responsibility within the family, following his brother's death. The disclosure of her husband's violence serves a narrative purpose in that context, evidencing and elaborating on the character and role of the son. Here, Rahmatullah is positioned as a heroic character within the restoration of the family narrative.

The second point is that the disclosure is extended, and perhaps even enabled, by the mother-in-law and sister-in-law. Throughout the interview, these women bring up subjects that Rahmatullah's mother has not previously disclosed, and extend her disclosure through their elaborations. The interviewer encourages this extended disclosure through her questions, as in the following extract:

Mother-in-law: This is my own house.
M: Yes, this is my mother-in-law's own house.[4] Because of family fights, they started living separately. After my son died, they came back to live with us. Since we are all alone after my son's death, they stayed back with us.
I: What happened? Why did they used to fight? What did they used to say?
M: Because of him.
I: Him means your husband?
M: Yes.
I: Fights were between him and your sisters in law?
M: With his mother, and sisters. He fights with everyone.
I: On what issues does he fight?
M: Just like that. When he says something, everyone must obey and do according to his wishes. If any one doesn't follow his orders, he fights.
I: When he fights with them, where would they go?

M: They never went anywhere. But the last time when he fought, he told them to move out. So they moved out.

I: Oh . . .

M: Yes that's how it is. They rented a house and stayed there.

This account emphasises the cohesiveness and supportiveness of the family other than the father. Thus, the mother-in-law and sister-in-law 'never went anywhere' until he forced them to move out, but in the family's time of extreme need – 'since we are all alone' – they returned: 'After my son died, they came back to live with us. Since we are all alone after son's death, they stayed back with us.' The disclosure of the father as problematic thus reinforces rather than disrupts the canonical narrative of the strong family and of strong women in the family. In this sense, the disclosure of domestic violence sheds new light on the mother's observation in Round 2: 'Everything and everybody else are fine, except him.'

Conclusions

In this chapter, I have focused on just one family case within the Young Lives dataset. In doing so, I risk reading out of context – not least as a UK researcher searching for narrative in Indian interviews, and reading in translation. However, in the analysis presented here, I have shown commonalities with themes identified through the wider cross-case analysis of Young Lives qualitative data in Andhra Pradesh (e.g. Morrow and Vennam 2009, Vennam and Komanduri 2009). These relate to Rahmatullah's increasing responsibilities within the family, especially following the major disruption of his brother's death, and in Rahmatullah's mother's experience of partner violence. Moreover, the aim of this case study analysis was to consider how a narrative analysis might provide insight into the meanings and effects of disclosures – through the stories told in interviews – because of its attention to absences, disruption and inconsistencies. I have presented contrasting examples of disclosure.

Rahmatullah's hesitant and managed revelations about his feelings about work and play appear difficult for him to reveal, and emerge in co-construction, through the interviewer's prompts and probes. They potentially disrupt the strong and responsible identity position – the 'good son', committed to his family – that he consistently foregrounds in all three rounds of interview. By contrast, Rahmatullah's mother's account of her husband's violence is at face value more conventionally recognisable as a 'disclosure' in the language of Western research ethics and social research. However, the story by which this information is revealed demonstrates the function of the disclosure as a narrative device, reinforcing the identities Rahmatullah's mother constructs for the rest of the family (including herself): the family as strong and self-sufficient, and Rahmatullah in particular as a key heroic figure in the restorative narrative developed following the family's bereavement. The bereavement itself – reflecting its enormous significance for the family – is told and retold through a series of small stories, with new elements revealed in each telling. Disclosure in this context has resonance with Bruner's (1991) account of narrative meaning making through story telling. In this light, Rahmatullah's mother's accounts can be seen as seeking to construct coherence, to make sense of a devastating and unexpected event.

As disclosures are made, in the telling of 'small stories', they illuminate the complexities, dynamism and tensions inherent in everyday family lives. By attending to the form of what is said, and to intentionality, within small stories and in their relationship to the progression of themes, it is possible to see how respondents construct individual and collective identities and how disclosures contribute to that construction. Disclosure, then, is not simply (nor only) about risk. In an interview context, as detailed here, disclosures can also be empowering – assisting the semantics and syntax of narrative to reinforce an identity position or strengthen a story. Participants are not merely passive respondents, but are also competent actors, revealing their everyday lives by telling the stories they wish to be told, in response and even in resistance to the interviewer's objectives and questioning.

Acknowledgements

The Family Lives and Environment project involves a team of researchers, including Ann Phoenix, Natasha Shukla and Catherine Walker, and members of the original Young Lives team, including Uma Vennam, Madhavi Latha, Virginia Morrow, Gina Crivello and Emma Wilson. The analysis presented here is my own, but has benefited from discussions with team members at all stages of the project to date. Particular thanks are due to the Young Lives team for such constructive advice on earlier drafts, and above all to Rahmatullah and his mother, for participating in Young Lives, and further agreeing that their data could be shared.

Notes

1. More information about NOVELLA (Narratives of Varied Everyday Lives and Linked Approaches) is available at www.novella.ac.uk.
2. For more information about the Young Lives qualitative longitudinal research, see Vennam and Komanduri 2009 and Crivello, Morrow and Wilson 2013, and www.younglives.org.uk/.
3. The pseudonym was assigned by Young Lives at the time of anonymisation of the transcripts. It is Young Lives protocol that the children have pseudonyms but other family members do not. Within the terms of our data access agreement with Young Lives, we have agreed to use only the assigned pseudonyms, and not to create additional pseudonyms, because of the risk of applying real names to family members without realising this. Hence we have not used a pseudonym for Rahmatullah's mother.
4. In Indian culture, including in Indian Muslim culture, it is common for a woman to live with her husband's family after marriage.

3 Being HIV positive

A phenomenology of HIV disclosure in Swaziland

Robin Root

Many modes of individual and social suffering inhere in experiences of HIV/AIDS. The specific modes I describe in this chapter are experienced among people living with HIV/AIDS (PLWHA) in the Kingdom of Swaziland. Once known as the Switzerland of southern Africa for its verdant, mountainous landscape and safe-haven status for foreign investments (Welz 2013), Swaziland is perhaps better known now as the last absolute monarchy in Africa and because it has the highest HIV/AIDS rates in the world. A confluence of political-economic, environmental and syndemic processes (Stringer, Thomas, and Twyman 2007) currently imperils the lives and livelihoods of much of the population. Approximately 45% of Swazi children are deemed orphaned and vulnerable (Joint United Nations Programme on HIV/AIDS [UNAIDS] 2012). HIV prevalence among young women age 15–24 (15.3%) is more than twice as high as that among young men (6.3%) (UNAIDS 2013: 101) and peaks shortly thereafter between ages 25 and 29 (49%). Men's rates peak between ages 35 and 39 (45%), a decade later than women's rates, which some scholars argue is evidence of women's greater vulnerabilities (Leclerc-Madlala 2008, Shannon et al. 2012). The multi-factorial violence suffered by the entirety of the Swazi social body is reflected in the nation's plummeting life expectancy, from 61 years to 32 years between 2000 and 2009 (Integrated Regional Information Networks [IRIN] 2009).

Yet recent progress suggests that large investments in HIV/AIDS programming may be paying off. In 2012, Swaziland successfully exceeded the United Nations General Assembly Special Session target of ensuring that at least 80% of HIV positive individuals needing antiretroviral treatment (ART/ARVs) were receiving it (Centres for Disease Control 2012). A decline in AIDS-related mortality has helped trend the average life expectancy upward to 50 years (World Health Organization [WHO] 2013). Treatment to prevent mother-to-child transmission (PTCMT) reached 95%, among the highest coverage rates in the sub-Saharan region (WHO 2013). Despite these advances, however, HIV disclosure in Swaziland, as elsewhere, can have serious ramifications for the individual disclosing and those with whom the disclosure is shared. For over three decades, HIV/AIDS research has remained primarily a bioscientific enterprise (MacQueen 2011, Adam 2011,

Kippax 2012). As a result, HIV disclosure studies have focused on important programmatic concerns, such as disclosure to sexual partners (Simoni and Pantalone 2004) and correlations with treatment uptake (Waddell and Messeri 2006). Although most of this research has focused on populations in the global North, an expanding literature on HIV disclosure in Africa is similarly aimed at strengthening HIV counselling and prevention. Studies have reported correlations between disclosure and sexual practices (Olley, Seedat and Stein 2004); disclosure rates, barriers and outcomes (Medley et al. 2004); psychosocial implications (Santamaria et al. 2011); factors associated with self-disclosure (Osinde, Kakaire and Kaye 2012); provider-initiated testing and disclosure rates (Kiene et al. 2010); and the effects of treatment on disclosure (Skogmar et al. 2006). Miller's and Rubin's qualitative study of HIV disclosure in Kenya (2007) was unique in conceptualising HIV disclosure not only as a behaviour but a culturally mediated phenomenon. By nesting disclosure within the communal social networks characteristic of much of Africa, the authors identified indirect communication, use of an intermediary, and church pastors as distinctive features of HIV disclosure that have been largely overlooked by conventional dyadic models focused on disclosure to sexual partners.

Recognising that individuals disclose for different reasons (Chaudoir and Fisher 2010), researchers have described disclosure motivations as either voluntary or without consent, where voluntary is further distinguished in terms of whether it was the person's will to disclose or because the individual felt compelled to do so (Chandra et al. 2003). Phenomenological anthropology (Marshall 1992, Kaufman 1988, Lopez and Willis 2004) may offer a more comprehensive understanding of disclosure through how its different meanings are produced, transformed and experienced by individuals within and across cultural settings (cf. Irving 2011, Rouleau, Côté and Cara 2012). Critical phenomenology is a particularly fitting lens for its perspective on both structural and cultural processes that influence experiences of HIV disclosure. One example of such an approach was Moses's and Tomlinson's study of women's HIV disclosure in Ethiopia, which portrayed disclosure as a fluid experience that accrued different meanings in different relationships over time (2012).

A culturally situated analysis of disclosure is integral to understanding HIV positivity more broadly, since the phenomenology of illness results 'not only from the experience of bodily disruption but from the effort to articulate that disruption' to others (Becker 2004: 129–30). In this chapter, I draw upon data from a medical anthropological project to explore the articulation of 'bodily disruption' caused by HIV infection in the form of HIV disclosure. Over the course of the project, detailed below, participants provided compelling accounts of the contextual features and significance of social relationships in shaping identity and strategies for survival, central to which was disclosure of one's HIV positive status to others. To generate phenomenological insights into HIV disclosure, I conducted an inductive and interpretive analysis of diverse qualitative data that suggested three entwined themes. These were (1) felt stigma as an embodied process that mediated experiences of HIV disclosure; (2) the role of social settings and reflexivity in disclosure decision making; and (3) the significance of antiretroviral treatment on HIV disclosure experiences. Although the accounts explored here profile HIV disclosure in rural Swaziland, they are relevant to populations in many parts of Africa where HIV prevalence is high, gender inequalities and material poverty are stark, and where Christianity, in various forms, is a salient feature of social life.

Study setting: the Kingdom of Swaziland

Asked what Swaziland would look like in 15 years, a chief who I interviewed predicted that unless 'the whites or Americans find a way to heal this disease, there won't be a Swaziland'. Indeed, preliminary reports from the national census in 2007 stated that the country had 'lost' an estimated 300,000 individuals, or 30% of its projected population, mostly as a result of HIV/AIDS (Nolen 2007).

Whether AIDS remains an 'exceptional' disease, a term coined early on by gay rights activists to mobilise political support for AIDS funding in the West, has been strenuously debated (Whiteside and Smith 2009). Detractors of AIDS exceptionalism maintain that AIDS has siphoned off a dispro-portionate share of global health funding. However, according to the former executive director of the UNAIDS, exceptionalism still holds since AIDS 'has broken with the general pattern of diseases and natural disasters, which usually create their own brutal equilibrium, eventually enabling societies to cope. AIDS . . . appears to be doing the opposite' (Piot 2005: 3). Excep-tionalism in Swaziland is starkly registered in its HIV epidemiology and poverty indices. Despite the country's lower middle income status (World Bank 2012), a majority of the population is unemployed (70%), living in chronic poverty (69.2%) and unable to meet basic food needs (66%) (International Fund for Agricultural Development 2013). Semi-subsistence agriculture remains a primary economic activity, but small-scale farming is a tenuous source of income and sustenance for most Swazis, a vast majority of whom reside on Swazi National Land (SNL). SNL is land held in trust by the King and has extremely low yields, in part because of insufficient public and private sector investments. By contrast, Title Deed Land, which is often the most arable, utilises 97% of the country's irrigated water and benefits from large-scale commercial agricultural investments (Manyatsi 2005). As a result, rural impoverishment has made threadbare the intrinsic social safety nets historically provided by extended families to its vulnerable members.

Politically, Swazi tradition, law and custom are enshrined in the country's constitution 'as pillars of the monarchy' (Commonwealth Local Govern-ment Forum [n.d.]: 207). The King (*iNgwenyama*) and Queen Mother (*iNdlovukazi*) preside at the helm of the Swazi monarchy and are central to the country's social organisation, policy formulation and ethnic identity. The current monarch, King Mswati III, was commended by global health agencies in 1999 for exercising his expansive powers when he declared AIDS in Swaziland a national disaster. In 2001, by invoking the *umchwaso* chastity rule banning sexual relations by and with girls under age 18, he conceded that culture could play an important role in shaping the epidemic, especially for young women. However, he breached his own ban just a few days later by taking a 17-year-old girl as his seventh wife (and fining himself one cow). Doing so enacted his monarchial prerogatives and, according to some observers, reinforced cultural practices of male sexual entitlement that conflicted with HIV prevention strategies.

From its inception, the AIDS epidemic has made it apparent that public health is a political enterprise. In Swaziland, this axiom presents unique challenges, primarily because it can be difficult for outsiders (non-Swazis) to grasp the deep cultural significance of the monarchy (Booth 1983). The King, with his influential Advisory Council (*liqoqo*), enacts power through the country's dual spheres of governance whose representatives pledge him unwavering loyalty and allegiance. The first sphere, the *tinkhundla*, is a patchwork of 55 constituencies that administer local government. Decentralising HIV/AIDS program management through the *tinkhundla* is an important component of the government's most recent strategic plan (Kingdom of Swaziland 2012). The second sphere, the *umphakatsi*, is comprised of 385 chiefdoms whose leaders and councils are the organising principle of sociopolitical life at the most local level (Green et al. 2009). The constitution describes the customary roles of the chief (*sikhulu/tikhulu*) as 'a symbol of unity and a father of the community' as well as the 'footstool' of the King through whom the King rules (Government of Swaziland [n.d.]: Chapter IV). Chiefs' gatekeeping roles were evident in the operations of a church-run home-based care organisation that I researched, as the group was obliged to secure chiefs' approval before providing services to the 22 communities where it operated.

Social identities and relationships in Swaziland are shaped as much by religious beliefs and affiliations as by one's place in the Swazi polity. Approximately 90% of the population identifies as Christian, a category that includes a wide range of pedagogies and practices (US Department of State 2008). From one-room wattle and daub to expansive concrete structures, churches are ubiquitous features of the country's physical and social landscape. Church participation is especially important for Swazi women. Across much of Africa, church networks often provide the only form of non-kin female association (Taylor 2006). The dissemination of Christianity in Swaziland reportedly began with the arrival of two German missionaries in 1844. Currently, a plurality of Christian denominations spans eight loosely bound categories: Zionist, Evangelical, Mainline, Pentecostal, Independent, Roman Catholic, other and unknown (Pan African Christian AIDS Network 2008).

Three national ecumenical bodies – the Council of Swaziland Churches, the League of African Churches, and the Swaziland Conference of Churches – provide leadership to their constituent denominations.

Diverse Christian meanings infuse matters of governance as well as medicine in Swaziland to produce a dynamic ideological saturation of social life. Despite longstanding criticism by AIDS activists in the global North, faith-based responses in many parts of Africa have demonstrated their 'exceptional' roles in addressing HIV/AIDS (Vitillo 2009: 77). A surplus of religious capital has been conceptualised as a health asset (African Religious Health Assets Program 2006) and helps to explain how religious places, discourses and social networks figure prominently in many Swazis' experiences of HIV/AIDS, including disclosure. In Swaziland, there exists approximately one church for every 200 Swazis versus one clinic per 6,451 persons. With a pastor for every local congregation, the ratio of religious leaders to medical staff is equally pronounced: 50 pastors versus two doctors per 10,000 Swazis. The Swaziland National Church Forum, an umbrella entity that has coordinated church responses to the epidemic since 1998, denounced HIV stigma a decade before the government did the same, earning it a 'best practices' profile by UNAIDS in 2006 (Swaziland Ministry of Health and Social Welfare 2008).

The project

The project upon which this chapter is based was designed to explore the nexus of culture, economy and epidemiology that gives HIV/AIDS its lived significance in Swaziland. The framing goal of the project was to evince a more nuanced understanding of HIV positivity by exploring felt stigma, religiosity, social networks, poverty and HIV practices, including disclosure. In this chapter, I theorise inductively from qualitative data as a method of apprehending the meanings of HIV disclosure for PLWHA. Purposive sampling strategies of HIV positive and church attending individuals generated mostly female respondents; across Africa, congregations are often comprised predominantly of women (Taylor 2006: 16) and, in Swaziland, women are more likely to have tested for HIV and retrieved their test results than men (Kingdom of Swaziland 2012: 8). Having knowledge of their HIV status, therefore, women were also more likely to face the challenges of disclosure.

The first of the project's five study phases began in Hhohho, the northernmost of Swaziland's four administrative regions. Residing with a Swazi family in a rural area, I conducted a 50-household questionnaire to deepen my understanding of household perceptions and experiences of rural poverty and HIV/AIDS. I also interviewed traditional healers, pastors, an HIV support group leader and a medical doctor at the regional health centre that had initiated free ART rollout six months earlier. By the end of this first phase, accounts of PLWHA and other participants pointed to moralistic discourses of HIV/AIDS and to religious sentiment as important domains for further investigation.

Walking the area's serpentine paths through meadows of dry winter grasslands, I witnessed the formalised etiquette of casual greetings between passers-by. Except for the ubiquitous crow of hens and roosters, rural Swaziland felt preternaturally quiet. The household questionnaire was conducted on grass mats or upturned buckets in dusty courtyards. Household is to some extent, however, a misnomer. Rural Swazis reside on what are known as homesteads (*umuti*), extended family compounds or, as Leliveld argues, a kin-based solidarity group (1994).

Historically, patrilocal and polygynous marriage practices expanded the number of rondavels on a homestead, since each wife, for whom brideprice (*lobola*) was paid in the form of cattle, was provided with a rondavel. The eldest son traditionally served as guardian and headman (*umnumzane*) (Patricks 2000). The living and the dead converged in and around the homestead *sibaya*, or cattle-byre, an open-air enclosure having both practical purposes and sacred meanings, where prayer and ancestor worship spanned both (Kuper 1980: 19). Traditionally, a family homestead included fenced fields where livestock, mostly cattle and fowl, were housed and smallholder crops (such as cotton or corn) cultivated. Homesteads remain the warp and weave of Swazi society, but their human and material resources have become severely depleted as a result of sickness and death, out-migration and economic degradation. As a result, homesteads often appeared sparsely populated, run down and lacking sufficient resources to maintain viable subsistence based households.

In 2006, I returned to the same community to investigate HIV stigma and disclosure in church settings (Root 2009, 2010). The semi-structured questionnaire was conducted in a small consultation room at the regional health centre located on a hill approximately 100 metres from a freshly paved road. Just beyond the main building was the health centre morgue. I was told that the concrete ramp leading from the building to the morgue had recently been expanded into a 'highway'. Outside the interview room, the waiting area was abuzz with a few dozen patients seated on concrete benches waiting to be tested and counselled. Wednesdays were designated medication refill days. On occasion, gospel hymns were audible from the other side of the closed door and a burst of laughter would ring out. The health centre emerged as one of the few places where individuals had no need to disclose. Their HIV positive status was a given. In an interview, an HIV testing counsellor said that an informal support group was taking shape, meeting under a tree on the health centre grounds to swap stories and share tips. At this point, ART had been available in the community for about 17 months. With more individuals on treatment, the general mood of the community felt considerably elevated from a year earlier, and HIV positive individuals who had been disabled with extreme sickness appeared healthier and invigorated.

During the third phase, I interviewed pastors around the country to explore their perceptions of the epidemic's impact on individuals, households and communities, and the contemporary roles of religion and religious leadership in times of crisis in Swaziland. During phases 4 and 5 in 2009 and 2011, I extended these lines of inquiry in the southern Shiselweni region, the most remote and least resourced in terms of government and international agency assistance. Because governments across much of Africa rely increasingly on home-based care to deliver HIV/AIDS services, my aim in researching the church-run Shiselweni Home-based Care organisation (SHBC) was to better understand the roles of religion and home-based care for individuals and communities hard hit by AIDS (Root 2011, Root and Van Wyngaard 2011). A South African pastor formed the SHBC in 2006 with 36 volunteers who responded to his call to assist the many individuals who were unwell in their communities. By 2011, 600 care supporters tended to 2,500 clients across 22 communities. Sporting mustard yellow jerseys with their organisation's motto 'To Become the Hands and Feet of Christ' across the back, the SHBC care supporters operated independently from the formal health system, although they regularly referred and escorted clients to clinics and spoke with health staff about the medical needs of specific clients.

Embodying disclosure: stigma, body, person

Anxieties over HIV stigma are paramount features of HIV disclosure, so much so that disclosure often functions as a 'proxy measure' for stigma (Obermeyer et al. 2011: 1015). The negative synergies of stigma and disclosure were evident in Greef's and colleagues' study of HIV stigma in five African countries, including Swaziland, where disclosure emerged as 'a spontaneous additional theme' reported by participants (2008: 311–12). A phenomenological study of HIV disclosure therefore requires consideration of the many permutations of HIV stigma that figure in being HIV positive and disclosing. Theories and frameworks for explaining HIV stigma are numerous, differentiated by their emphasis on structural (Parker and Aggleton 2003, Link and Phelan 2001), cultural (Ogden and Nyblade 2005, Holzemer et al. 2007) and socio-psychological features (Earnshaw and Chaudoir 2009, Deacon 2006, Campbell and Deacon 2006).

The notion of stigma as a moral process may be especially productive because HIV disclosure requires that each party wrestle with its impact on 'what matters most' to discloser and interlocutor alike (Yang et al. 2007: 1528). Core values of 'what matters most' in Swaziland largely concern the affective and material viability of social relationships with both living persons and ancestral spirits. According to anthropologist Hilda Kuper, a '[Swazi] person is a meeting point of identities – the identity of siblings, the identity of lineage, the identity of the age group' (1986 [1963]: 59). The convergence of multiple identities on the individual person means that survival of body and self hinge on the responses of multiple and overlapping social networks to one's disclosure. This ongoing dialectic of competing claims on core social values shaped the everyday lives of individuals as they deliberated whether, how and to whom to disclose their HIV positive status. An ideology of kin, closeness and support imbues food, for example, with symbolic power. More than a physical place or even a social group, homesteads are the most culturally valued institution for 'assuring [the Swazi's] birthright to support and sustenance from the land and other wealth of the Swazi nation' (Ngubane 1983: 10). The ideology of birthright and sustenance on/from one's homestead was a discrete feature of many participants' disclosure experiences. A 58-year-old woman described how her adult children 'shocked' and 'stigmatised' her by refusing to share food with her after she disclosed to them. Expressing stigma by withholding food demonstrated how 'stigma is not just a discursive or interpretive process, but a fully embodied, physical, and affective process that takes place in the posture, positioning, and sociality of the sufferer' (Yang et al. 2007: 1530). Withholding sustenance therefore expressed the children's moralistic judgement that positive HIV status had stripped their mother of legitimate social status. She was no longer a person. Ruel has written about the idea of the shadow as 'the lively counterpart' in many African societies to the Western concept of a person (1993). In Swaziland, he writes, this shadow is 'dependent for its vitality upon his active movement and relationship to others – his identity as represented by his interaction with others' (Ruel 1993: 103–4). Physically weakened by HIV/AIDS, a disease of the presumptively sexually immoral or transgressive, an HIV positive person may become vulnerable to an ever-diminishing number and quality of social interactions. The cumulative effect was a diminishment of that individual's personhood by diminishing their 'shadow'. According to a young male participant, without employment, your life becomes – he pincered his index finger to his thumb – 'this small'. A recent job offer at a sugar manufacturing facility was revoked after a fellow community member informed management that he was HIV positive.

To replace the loss of vital social relationships, care supporters with the SHBC organisation established new modes of sociality and drew upon discourses of Christian love to constitute new modes of HIV personhood. In the case of the mother above, the participant's care supporter counselled her adult children on the importance of providing her with proper nutrition and compassion. Asked whether there were religious aspects to the care she received from the SHBC, the woman described how the care supporter recited biblical verses about Job's tribulations to remind her that even though her children stigmatised her, God's love was ever present. The care supporter's dual intervention was transformative. One of the children began tending to her mother's needs and the care supporter's spiritual counselling recast the woman's shamed sense of self, enlarging her shadow and putting it in sharp relief. The participant said she no longer felt like committing suicide.

HIV stigma continues to be a pervasive feature of HIV/AIDS in Swaziland that threatens to undermine HIV/AIDS programming (Dlamini et al. 2009, Zamberia 2011, Joint United Nations Programme on HIV/AIDS 2012). In a national report of HIV stigma among PLWHA in Swaziland, 45% of respondents indicated that they were unwilling to go to the clinic for ARVs because of concerns that doing so would alert others to their positive status (IRIN 2012). Early in the project, I spoke with a woman in her fifties who, despite her emaciated body, was voluble about being HIV positive. Both she and her husband had tested positive, but they could only afford treatment for him at a government hospital. I returned to her homestead the following day to tell her about the free ART recently made available at the health centre only a few kilometers away. She seemed irked by this information and informed my interpreter that she was aware of the medicines, but that the nurses had gossiped about her status when she went there to test, so she was reluctant to return. (On a return trip a year later, the woman appeared to be in strong form as she hauled bales of hay onto a flatbed.)

In addition to gossip, participants reported Swazi epithets that referenced a person with HIV: they were a walking coffin, keys to the mortuary, or had one foot in the grave. The sick body was indexed as vulnerable, dangerous and shameful in other ways as well. A 33-year-old woman, unmarried with six children, imagined that if she disclosed to her congregation, church women whom she'd witnessed provide bananas and oranges to the sick might do the same for her. She was afraid to do so, however, because some people, 'if you tell them, they tend to laugh at you, and that can destroy you and make you more sick'. Her multiple statuses – unwell, female, poor – framed her experience of her body as an object in need, the voicing of which risked exacerbating her sickness and harming her body further.

Conceptually, the illness experience is predicated on individuals' narration of their pain and suffering as a means for others to access those meanings (Kleinman 1988: 5). However, if illness talk is occluded in high stigma settings, as HIV/AIDS often is, the concept of the illness experience is inadequate to explicating a key aspect of being positive: speaking one's HIV positive status. Some participants disclosed their status to me by answering the question, 'How is your health?' with the response that they were on 'the blue pills', rather than telling me directly they were HIV positive or had AIDS. It was common knowledge that the blue pills were antiretrovirals. Later in the conversation, the term HIV or 'the body's soldiers', a term used at clinics to explain CD4 counts as measures of immune system health, would be introduced into our conversation. Participants also asserted that AIDS was rampant in Swaziland and that 'people are dying left and right'. But when asked whether AIDS was common around 'here', at which point I gestured to the environs where the participant and I were seated, the answer was often that it was not so common. HIV-related suffering was similarly displaced when pastors warned their congregations of 'the many diseases out there' and exhorted congregants to 'take care of themselves and others who are sick'. The referents of 'diseases', 'others' and 'sick' were presumed to be known and their meanings shared. They were, but the details of these conditions remained unspoken and unspecified.

Circumlocution around taboo diseases is common to many cultures, but the forms it takes varies. In Swaziland, children are socialised through riddles and verbal memory games (Kuper 1986 [1963]: 53), the resolution of which demonstrated intelligence and maturity. While there may not exist a direct line connecting riddles with circumlocutory discourses around HIV, the premise that there may be a way of talking of AIDS by talking around it offers one schema by which to grasp the idiosyncratic challenges in Swaziland, not only of disclosure as a discrete event but of its different meanings. Describing a method to represent ineffable experiences of sickness, Irving has called for an anthropology of interiority to theorise the inchoate negotiation of self and social relations among PLWHA in Uganda, emphasising:

> the often unvoiced but sometimes radical changes in being, belief, and perception that can occur while carrying out everyday, routine activities: changes in identity and body image; changes in people's aesthetic appreciation of time and existence; changes in preexisting practices and religious beliefs; changes in the type of imaginary worlds people inhabit in relation to material surroundings; and changes in the character and meaning of everyday social roles and interactions while experiencing decline, entering a new existential territory, or attempting to reclaim life.
>
> (Irving 2011: 26–7)

According to Rapport, interiority describes the 'continual conversation one has with oneself . . . how individual consciousness feels in the everyday and is immanent in social life' (2008: 331). To access aspects of that conversation and consciousness, I asked people in Swaziland to describe their rationales for disclosing or not disclosing their HIV status in church settings. Responses exteriorised an inner dialogue that envisaged the potential advantages and pitfalls of doing so. Many participants who had not disclosed their HIV positive status to fellow congregants or their pastors often reflected on their deep wish to do so, in part to secure spiritual, emotional and material support. For example, intensified food needs, disabling sickness and side effects from medications meant asking others for assistance, which required some form of disclosure. People longed also for the subjective sense and socially constructed quality of 'courage' they witnessed being attributed to those who did share knowledge of their HIV positive status with fellow church members. Thus, while gossiping and other stigmatising modes functioned to deter HIV disclosure, the possibility of assistance and establishing a new sense of self, noteworthy for its courage, served as incentives.

The notion of interiority as an 'unvoiced discourse' that irrupts as breaches of public conventions (Rapport 2008: 338) helps to explicate the meanings of disclosure. After she cut her finger during a church project, a 50-year-old woman disclosed her HIV positive status when she warned others not to touch her blood and requested a Band-Aid. She recalled how her disclosure was met with incredulous laughter. Surely, no one would publicly declare something as shameful as being HIV positive. She repeated herself. Their response, she recalled, was to do nothing. The initial laughter and subsequent silence in the face of her disclosure reflected, in her view, that 'Swazis are hard like stones. They do not want to know or tell the truth.' She was different, she explained. God had helped her not to be a stone. He gave her courage to speak her truth. Interviewed again one year later, the woman said that her fellow parishioners treated her well. Only one individual had attempted to silence her disclosure post factum, telling her 'It was not good to tell people you are HIV-positive.' The participant countered that her disclosure was the right thing to do as it might help others similarly afflicted to seek help, therefore establishing a higher moral ground as a result of being HIV positive.

Stigma is often codified in 'forms of social prejudice and power' (Deacon 2006: 421). These forms may affect disclosure decisions, including notification of sexual partners. One HIV counsellor cited polygamy (*sitsembu*) as among the health centre's most significant challenges. In Swaziland, polygynous marital arrangements allow a man to take multiple wives provided that he can, in principle, provide equally for each woman and her offspring. Status accrues to the man with many wives (Buseh et al. 2002). Polygyny within the Swazi patriarchal framework includes other cultural practices which some argue may accelerate the spread of HIV (United Nations Development Programme 2008). These include widow inheritance (*kungena*), whereby a widow is married to her dead husband's brother after a two-year mourning period (*kuzila*); sexual access to a wife's younger sister for childbearing if a wife is infertile (*kuhlanta*); and courtship of a wife's younger sister, which tends nowadays to include sexual relations (*kulamuta*) (Zwane 2006). In a report on an initiative to grant women the right to refuse participation in a range of customary practices such as these, a Swazi judge argued that 'animals have more rights and freedoms than a woman here' (cited in Lucas 2005: 62). Detailing the challenges these sociocultural conditions posed for testing and counselling, the same clinic counsellor described how wives drew on a discourse of empowerment and individual bodily concern to resist pressures to disclose, stating that they were responsible only for their own health:

> Counselors will ask a woman: 'What did you do, did you communicate this with your sisters [co-wives] and your husband?' The woman says, 'Nope, that's none of their business. I'm concentrating on my health.'

Women's decisions not to disclose to each member of a polygynous marriage posed a complex and dangerous public health dilemma. Ideally, each member (and their children) of the sexual network would be tested and, if necessary, placed on treatment, and all sexual relations would require condom usage to prevent further viral risk and exposure. Women's unwillingness to disclose left them open to criticism and blame for failing to extend the public health project into the domestic space – the homestead. Women's seeming lack of compliance was, to some extent, an act of defiance against marital power structures and public health agendas alike. In the interview, the counsellor continued:

Can you imagine the trouble, the problem that she is doing to the family, because she will not communicate this to the husband? And then, if you go and have sex there without a condom, imagine the resistance for the husband and the others? . . . You're just wasting [the medications] and we tell them, 'If you feel you just want to go back there and have fun, forget about the tabs. Once you think you're ready, then you can come back.' . . . You know, we hear them talking; like, you hear 'Oh, I don't mind if he doesn't want to come in to test. I will come here to test. I will come here and take my test and continue to take my drugs . . . Even if they die, I'm not interested.' . . . They feel as long as they're taking the drugs, they're safe.

On occasion, interviews became interventions, which shed a different light on the complex clinical and sociocultural dynamics of HIV positivity in marital life. An HIV positive widow whom I had interviewed a year earlier expressed confusion over the rules and risks of ART adherence, disclosure, and widow inheritance. She said she was suffering from herpes zoster, an opportunistic infection, across her chest that was painful. At the time, public health campaigns were emphasising the risks of failed adherence, which led the woman to wonder which risk was greater: missed medications (she lived far from the health centre and transport was costly) or no medication at all. She also asked whether she should disclose her HIV status to her brother-in-law, a man to whom she might be married after two years mourning in accordance with the custom of widow inheritance (*kungena*). Cognisant of the complex ethics of counselling her, my Swazi interpreter and I brought her to the health centre for treatment and counselling.

Asked how she dealt with HIV/AIDS in her own congregation, an elderly female pastor, whose own adult children, she said, had AIDS, explained how she uses the metaphor of a shedding snake to teach people not to stigmatise those with HIV: 'You have a life and future,' she tells her parishioners. 'A snake moves forward; a snake does not go back and retrieve its old skin. It sheds its skin. Forget about the old skin. We must leave behind the stigmatising attitude like a snake leaves behind its old skin. People must change their stigmatising behaviour; no matter how the person got the HIV, we're all affected.' Given pervasive HIV stigma, Ntsimane (2006) advocated the importance of creating safe spaces for self-disclosure. Towards that end, SHBC care supporters found themselves increasingly playing the role of an intermediary, or a disclosure broker, helping clients to imagine and enact HIV disclosure to appropriate others (Root and Van Wyngaard 2011). Disclosure counselling was available at health clinics, but these resources were not readily accessible: transport was costly and some individuals were too ill to travel. Moreover, as one participant observed, contrasting SHBC care supporters with health centre staff, the latter had provided her with 'full counselling' but the 'care supporters are nearer to us each and every day. They are close to us. And we are open to speak to the care supporter about things that we are afraid to speak to the nurses about.'

Stigma and shame exerted their effects on disclosure decision-making in part by rendering the HIV body a cultural object for amplification and concealment (Csordas 1990: 34). When people feared a person's body and undertook practices to avoid proximity, the HIV positive body felt amplified by the projection of cultural symbols of danger, transgression and disease. Efforts to resist those projections might entail educating others about the nature of one's infection. A 23-year-old participant had disclosed to no one at church, having told only her family. One day a parishioner informed her that fellow congregants were scared that an infection on her face was contagious. She protested that her body had an inside and outside: 'This won't spread to anyone, because it's from the inside; it's just showing up that I've got something, so I have to go to the hospital and get this treated.' Fears of HIV/AIDS linked with perceptible infection on her face precipitated further body demarcation, as she observed that the person who customarily sat next to her had relocated to a different seat. Despite these derogations of her body and exclusion from a vital social network, she was considering disclosing to her pastor. He was able to give positive public meanings to her disclosure, evidenced by his calls for parishioners to care for and not stigmatise those who are 'sick'. She envisioned a scene where he would 'tell the whole congregation that so-and-so has got this problem, so if she's not around, maybe sick, we should pray for her.' In her imagined HIV disclosure, actuated through a religious leader, the absence of her feared body from church services would inspire concern rather than elicit dread from those in her presence.

Disclosure: managing speech and silence

Disclosure is synonymic with exposure, divulgence and revelation (Dictionary.com 2013). Each of these words is imbued with connotations of the secret rendered social and has elements of drama and performance. Chaudoir and colleagues define an HIV disclosure event 'as the verbal communication that occurs between a discloser and a confidant regarding the discloser's HIV positive status' (2011: 1620). In Swaziland, participants' experiences of identifying a confidant and subsequent disclosure varied by setting (e.g. home or church) and social position (e.g. sex/gender, marital status or age). Homesteads, as extended family compounds comprised of multiple dwellings, often constituted primary lifeworlds for PLWHA. Participants described a range of family reactions to their disclosure, from acceptance, encouragement and relief, to sadness, fear and rage. Articulating an HIV positive status could secure much needed support, but it might also disrupt social relationships. This might happen, for example, if prolonged sickness triggered a 'rupture of the rules of reciprocity that are the basis for social interactions' (Obermeyer et al. 2011: 1017). Among participants, reasons for not seeking family support fell into two categories that often overlapped: material and psychosocial. In the first, electing not to call upon family members was often a function of generalised poverty. 'They are poor like me and can't help,' explained a 42-year-old woman. If a participant did seek assistance, they might do so only once. 'I'm scared if I ask [my family] once,' said a 65-year-old woman, 'and then I ask again, I fear they will say I am a burden to them.'

A pivotal dimension of disclosure decision making was therefore an individual's expectation of how family members might react. One woman said she was thrown out of her family's home. Another woman recounted how her husband had encouraged her to be tested before they were married, because he had tested and learned that he was positive. She did so and found that she, too, was positive. His family confronted her as to why her husband had married her, as she was unable to have children (which they attributed to her having HIV). People seemed to attribute everything she did to her HIV status, which came to define her every action. If she was at the market buying fruits and vegetables, people said she was doing so because she is HIV positive; many government campaigns encourage HIV positive persons to eat healthily, especially lots of fruits and vegetables. If there was a social event and she said she could not eat beef, again they said it was because she was HIV positive.

Speaking one's status was to some extent a breach of propriety, where 'these supposed public acts may be reinterpreted as something other besides: moments where the private voice breaks the surface of conventional discourse' (Rapport 2008: 346). An elderly man, who said he was over 60, said his family laughed at him when he told them he had tested positive. They called him stupid for disclosing: this was something to be kept confidential. In contrast, the children of a 62-year-old woman told her, 'Ma, don't worry. You are a human being. We're there for you.' However, this same woman felt unable to tell her husband who had a drinking problem and with whom she did not share a bedroom. Some participants selectively indicated their status to individuals whose bodies they witnessed were deteriorating, recognising the signs and symptoms of possible HIV infection, hoping to encourage the person to seek testing and treatment. The study of Shamos and colleagues likewise found that HIV positive individuals were partly motivated by 'the desire to be helped, to protect others, to inform, and to inspire' (2009: 1682).

Church participation was important for many PLWHA. Participants had observed those who disclosed subsequently receiving assistance. Substantial anti-stigma and pro-care messages from their pastors made disclosure seem a desirable if daunting act. Church-based experiences of HIV/AIDS were also elicited in interviews with Swazi pastors. One young pastor's mother was a nurse and an HIV counsellor. His church sponsored health workshops once a year, at which attendees were counselled to disclose to someone if they were HIV positive, someone 'who they trust the most . . . because this has to be my secret and your secret. And the communication between me and you has to be our secret. I have to take care of your situation.' Disclosure was thus encouraged within the framework of a shared secret. Selecting an appropriate interlocutor was a high stakes endeavour: 'If the person receiving the secret conveys "disgust or a shame" . . . I am just killing you.' In other words, HIV disclosure was constructed as an embodied imperative because it may be the best, if riskiest, means of securing a caring relationship upon which survival and selfhood may depend.

Building rapport and creating safe places for individuals to decide whether to test, seek treatment and disclose were central aims of the SHBC. The group's care supporters selected their clients in part on the basis of how sick an individual appeared to be, or who, through word-of-mouth, was known to be extremely unwell. Many who were very sick fell out of view, removed from the public landscape by disability. Care supporters were not always certain of a client's HIV status at the outset of the care relationship, so they strategically guided early conversations to determine whether the person had been tested; if not, clients were encouraged to test for various infections and conditions to gain a more complete picture of the client's ill health and to normalise HIV testing. Clients emphasised the importance that a care supporter be a Christian. Because many Swazis identify as Christians, it is important to determine what participants meant when they invoked 'being Christian' in these instances: Christian was a discursive label often invoked to describe the nature of a person's heart rather than a denominational affiliation. A Christian care supporter thus was held to be more capable of compassion and more inclined to protect an individual's confidentiality than a non-Christian care supporter.

The impact of the special trust ascribed to Christian care supporters was evident in HIV testing and disclosure rates. Some 30% of participants reported that they sought testing following counselling by their care supporter; 25% said care supporters had been involved in their HIV disclosure to family or others. One care supporter recounted the story of an HIV positive husband and wife, who did not know of each other's positive status. One day, the husband, who was her client, told the care supporter that while he wanted to disclose, he was afraid his wife would leave him. The care supporter told the man, 'I have a plan.' She would bring a chicken to the couple's home on a Saturday night, and the three of them would chat and enjoy dinner together. When the moment seemed right, she recalled telling him, he could tell his wife. On the scheduled evening, at the anticipated moment, the husband initiated his disclosure: 'Now, my wife, what if I told you I'm HIV positive?' She answered that she would accept him, because after all, 'You are still a human being.' He told her of his HIV positive status. She, in turn, disclosed that she, too, was HIV positive. She left the room, returning with her handbag so that she could show him her medications. The husband went outdoors, and from beneath a tree, he dug up his own medications.

Culturally situated talk about HIV disclosure, religion and the formation of new social relationships opened up for examination and reflection deep-seated fears about other people knowing one's HIV positive status. By ensuring that prejudice and shame no longer monopolised conversations around HIV/AIDS, intra- or inter-subjectively, SHBC care supporters helped clients to navigate the insecurities and anxieties of disclosure and to experience a certain relief or liberation having done so. In the process, care supporters, clients and their families collectively authored an emerging discourse of being HIV positive and transforming the meanings and experiences of disclosure.

Disease chronicity: a lifetime of disclosure

HIV/AIDS has the potential to become a chronic condition among those with reliable access to life-extending medications and proper support. However, conventional notions of disease chronicity 'do not adequately capture life with HIV for most people' (Colvin 2011: 4). A key facet of this 'life with HIV' is that, over a lifetime, it will likely entail numerous disclosures of a condition seen as taboo and transgressive. Prior to ARVs, individuals would be housebound by sickness until death, diminishing the necessity and opportunities for disclosure. Now, with regained health, individuals on treatment have the option to move about the social world. Thus, with chronicity, disclosure becomes processual, subject to individuals' shifts in emotional, bodily, social, political and economic conditions. The result is an ongoing negotiation of body, self and identity. A central aim of a phenomenological agenda is to apprehend 'the subjectivity of human actors as it is shaped into, experienced and interpreted as an "objective reality"' (Knibbe and Versteeg 2008: 48). Rendering such private experiences as an objective reality for others to grasp was often challenging. For example, a 27-year-old participant said that when fellow church members learned that she was HIV positive, some ceased speaking with her. This was disconcerting, because her pastor had encouraged parishioners to 'take care of their neighbours, as that person may be bedridden and unable to retrieve their ARVs'. When parishioners did speak with her, she described how they recurrently required her to disclose: 'I've heard from so-and-so that you are HIV positive,' to which she would respond, 'Yes, I'm HIV positive.' Yet, she continued, after commencing ARVs, she appeared sufficiently healthy – 'back to her old self' – so that some parishioners resumed speaking to her as they had prior to her diagnosis, and opined that she was not HIV positive after all. Such claims called into question the 'objective reality' of HIV, effectively negating the woman's HIV status and subverting the fact of her self disclosure.

An individual's experience of coming to know HIV as an objective reality, which occurred in the provision of a test result, and the myriad emotions that accompanied diagnosis, were evident in the account of a 30-year-old woman who felt she needed a care supporter in her life to remind her of her infection. She needed to vigilantly tend to her body with ARVs. Consciousness of this reality appeared to fluctuate, posing a substantial risk to her fragile health: 'I don't understand things about the sickness. At times, I may think I'm not HIV positive and may want to stop ARVs, but the care supporters answer my questions.' By virtue of the care relationship, her supporters helped to constitute a subjective understanding of her body as HIV infected, a diagnosis that, at times, the participant was not certain was real.

A similar embodied disconnect was reported in a World Health Organization study of PLWHA's quality of life, where 'a conflict between actual and perceived body image [was] exacerbated by the phenomenology of the HIV infection' (2003: 350). Indeed, the dramatic reconstitutions of body and self that ARVs can materialise approximate the biblical:

> The narratives of chronic HIV infection and treatment . . . centre on an image of either a resurrected body (the 'Lazarus effect' of ART) or a vibrant, healthy body that never had to be resurrected (because of early treatment), a body that is strong and newly disciplined in maintaining treatment and lifestyle adherence, newly normalised as the sufferer . . . of just another chronic condition with no specified endpoint.
>
> (Colvin 2011: 4)

In some instances, disclosure was less about communicating an HIV positive status than struggling to persuade interlocutors of the veracity of a diagnosis. Conflicting perceptions of an improved bodily appearance could diminish the relief an individual might feel at no longer looking so sickly, when their sick body was an implicit disclosure of their condition. A 32-old-year woman described how a care supporter helped her to disclose to her family. The participant hoped that disclosure, with evidence of her body restored by ARVs, would prove the benefits of testing and treatment, which her sister refused to seek:

The care supporter helped me to tell my family, because my sister was also sick. I was afraid to tell her, because I thought she would say that I am laughing at her, or bluffing. So the care supporter advised me to make an example with my life. But my sister couldn't accept the [HIV] positive life, so she passed on [died].

Her family nonetheless refused to believe that she was HIV positive and distrusted her claim of the effectiveness of ARVs:

My [natal] family didn't believe I was being helped by the ARVs to get well. They said I was just telling stories. Since my sister died, [though], they try to believe me . . . I decided on my own to tell my in-laws that I am living positively. Even they don't believe I have HIV. My mother-in-law reminds me when to take the ARVs, but doesn't believe I have HIV.

The refusal of family members to believe that she was HIV positive inflicted a different kind of pain:

It hurts me a lot [that they do not believe me], because they're busy dying left and right, because they do not believe what I am saying. So I pray one day that they may accept that I am HIV positive.

In a similar manner, a 60-year-old male participant said family members initially threatened to kill him when he tried to explain CD4 counts. Because he suspected his brother had AIDS-related dementia, he felt compelled to disclose to encourage his brother to be tested and access treatment. Despite initial hostility, however, unlike the woman's sister above, the man's brother complied. Now, the participant said, his brother 'preaches the gospel to get tested'.

Perhaps the most salient instance of a phenomenology of disclosure occurred in an interview with an HIV positive pastor who had established two congregations in Swaziland after working in the mines in South Africa. There he experienced God exhort him to 'stop going underground' lest one day he fail to emerge alive. Heeding the call to establish a church, the pastor used his sermons to encourage HIV testing and ARV treatment, and hosted a monthly all-night vigil for one parishioner, an HIV positive man, to share his experiences publicly 'to teach us how to live with this virus'. Two or three men subsequently came forward and disclosed as well. The pastor desired deeply to tell his congregants of his own status and of his experience of ARVs, to use his body and authority to encourage them to seek testing and treatment 'because if you are counselling somebody, you're supposed to say, "Look at me, I have been through that."' But a clinic counsellor had advised him that, 'As you are a pastor, don't try to confess until the right times come', and he feared that to confess, to disclose, would cause congregants to 'run away' and the church to dissolve. He said he was waiting on God who was 'the only one who is going to give me the date . . . I'm still waiting for the right time.'

Conclusion

There is extensive suffering, personal and collective, as a result of HIV/AIDS, via its pathology and epidemiology, and its experience in a setting marked by multiple vulnerabilities. To examine local suffering and HIV/AIDS is to probe global processes of structural violence (Farmer 1999, Singer and Clair 2003), biomedical regimes of disease etiology and intervention (Bastos 1999), and cultural transformations in sentiments and personal relatedness that bear on quality of life and survival (Klaits 2010). The challenge for studying HIV disclosure is that in Swaziland, for many people, AIDS is a disease condition that cannot readily be spoken, for which there are no 'publicly accepted sets of meanings and symbols' (Obeyeskere 1985: 147).

The meanings of HIV disclosure in Swaziland relate to the lived nexus of colonial history, global political economy, epidemiology and reification of tradition in Swazi discourses. For its focus on the embodied mediation of historical, material and sociocultural processes, the phenomenological approach used in this chapter helped to apprehend diverse aspects of being HIV positive, including of disclosure. A next generation phenomenological question would be 'whether, and how, a critique of political and socio-economic circumstances can be formulated by focusing on experience and embodiment' (Knibbe and Versteeg 2008: 59). These linkages are important conceptually and programmatically. First, a phenomenological frame recasts the 'neo-liberal rational [subject]' too often reified in health promotion models as one who is somehow *sui generis* to history and the culture-specific lifeways that characterise a group of people (Kippax 2012: 6). Instead, individuals inhabit a world that they did not create, but to which they are subject (Miller 1982: 204). Hickel's political-economic analysis of AIDS in Swaziland describes a 'world' of pathological privilege and inequality sourced from and sustained by neoliberal policies that consolidate the interests of a very few at the expense of the population (2012: 517). Hickel intimates a critical phenomenology of HIV infection, noting as one conse-quence of the neoliberal agenda a 'western biomedical paradigm that fetishises the individual as the locus of agency and responsibility and assumes rigid distinctions between individual bodies and the broader social world' (2012: 515). Further, anthropological engagement with bodies in distress is a source of essential insight into the impact of the expanded ARV roll-out, as conventional discourses of chronicity may limit a deeper understanding of how HIV illness is experienced by individuals in resource poor settings (Colvin 2011: 5).

In their study of HIV disclosure in South Africa, Norman and colleagues found that 'civil society movements surrounding HIV/AIDS [have] fostered the transformation of the stigma and marginalisation previously associated with HIV/AIDS into new forms of belonging, and perhaps ultimately, citizenship in the HIV-positive economy' (2007: 1780). They argue that these new modes of belonging could facilitate 'a virtuous cycle' of disclosure, benefiting individuals and entire societies. A phenomenological study of HIV disclosure must concern itself, therefore, with a political economy of infection and a moral economy of care. In the absence of progress in the former, the burden has fallen on the latter to ensure some measure of social cohesion and continuity in the lives of those afflicted. As the accounts provided in this chapter indicate, SHBC care supporters' relationships with HIV positive individuals and their families were pivotal in making biomedical interventions actionable. They resurrected individuals' sense of personhood, and rendered HIV/AIDS an effable condition, so saving and restoring many lives. The ripple effects of such activism may not reach economic roundtables. However, these relationships, which in public health parlance would be termed interventions, could well translate into transformative political actions. As one mode of Swazi civic engagement and spanning 2,500 sq km, the SHBC organisation has given voice to the social suffering of a majority who, individually, struggle to speak their pain and to disclose.

Acknowledgements

I extend my heartfelt thanks to the individuals and organisations, especially Arnau Van Wyngaard, Shorty Khumalo and the care supporters and clients of the Shiselweni Reformed Home-based Care Organisation. I am also grateful to Alan Whiteside, Executive Director of the Health Economics and HIV/AIDS Research Division (HEARD), at the University of KwaZulu-Natal, for its research support. The Research Foundation of the City University of New York has been a sponsor of the project from its inception.

4 Emotional talk

Depression, diagnosis and disclosure

Renata Kokanovic and Brigid Philip

For many of us, telling others about our emotional ups and downs – that is, disclosing – is an everyday practice. We talk to friends, family members, even colleagues and friendly strangers about our daily worries, pain, anguish and generally unpleasant emotions and moods, as well as our joys, triumphs and pleasant experiences. Studies of lay understandings of emotions reveal a widespread belief that emotional disclosures to supportive friends and family members help people to deal with pain and adversity, maintain emotional health, and build strong personal relationships (Pollock 2009). Yet many people also disclose their emotional distress to medical practitioners, and on the basis of these disclosures, many are diagnosed with depression and/or prescribed antidepressant medication (Pollack 2007, Rogers et al. 2001). The World Health Organization (WHO 2008) estimates that almost 100 million people are diagnosed with depression globally. In Australia, where the authors of this chapter reside, most prescriptions for mental-health related illnesses are for antidepressants, with approximately 13 million scripts written each year, a significant number in a country of roughly 22.63 million people (ABS 2007).

The reasons for the increasing trend towards disclosing emotional distress to medical practitioners are myriad and complex. Jacob (2006) has argued that the progressive medicalisation of emotional distress in recent decades, accompanied by media reports about the so-called depression 'epidemic', may have contributed to increasing numbers of people consulting medical practitioners about emotional problems. Others have argued that the aggressive marketing of psycho-pharmaceuticals has created a new relationship between contemporary subjects and prescription drugs whereby people start to question the need for drugs such as antidepressants in their own lives (Jenkins 2011: 20). Depression has also been the subject of widespread online mental health literacy campaigns in countries such as Australia, which encourage people to disclose their depressive 'symptoms' to their medical practitioners so that they can gain access to appropriate treatment, usually antidepressants (see www.beyondblue.org.au). In this context, people experiencing emotional distress may eventually come to question whether they have depression, whether they need antidepressants, and whether they should disclose feelings of distress to their doctor in order to be medically diagnosed and treated.

For people who are diagnosed or treated for depression, decisions arise about whether or not to disclose their diagnosis or antidepressant treatment to members of their social network. Some people may have already disclosed their feelings to a partner or close friend before consulting a doctor. In these relationships there may be no decision to disclose the diagnosis as such, as confidants are intimately involved in the diagnostic process (Flaherty, Pleloran and Browner, this volume). In many relationships, however, the person diagnosed with depression will need to decide whether to tell others of the diagnosis, and, if so, whom to disclose to, how and when. Media stories about celebrity disclosures tend to frame disclosure of a depression diagnosis in positive terms. These dominant cultural narratives emphasise the personal benefits of disclosure in terms of relieving the burden of keeping a secret and being true to oneself (Blackman 2007). Furthermore, celebrities who publicly disclose a diagnosis of depression are often praised for raising public awareness and de-stigmatising mental illness (Blackman 2007). The recent emergence of the mental health recovery movement also emphasises the benefits of sharing personal stories of mental illness as a means to challenge negative stereotypes (Ridge and Ziebland 2012: 741). Similarly, most of the medical and psychological literature emphasises the positive impacts of disclosing one's diagnosis to others as a means to access medical care, combat stigma, gain social support and involve family and friends in treatment and recovery (see Norman et al. 2010, Bos et al. 2009, Corrigan et al. 2004, Corrigan and Matthews 2004, Scambler 2004). However, recent research about contested illnesses, such as chronic fatigue syndrome (Dickson et al. 2007, Dummit 2006), fibromyalgia syndrome (Barker 2011), borderline personality disorder (Koehne et al. 2012) and phobias (Davidson 2005), reveals that disclosure decisions can be highly problematic for people who have been diagnosed. According to these studies, disclosing a contested diagnosis can erode people's sense of authenticity, undermine the legitimacy of their illness experience, and negatively impact on personal and professional relationships.

Depression has been described as a contested illness, that is, 'an illness that is framed as difficult, psychosomatic, or even non-existent by researchers, health practitioners, and policy makers operating within conventional paradigms of knowledge' (Moss and Teghtsoonian 2008: 7, see also Kokanovic et al. 2012). Within the medical profession, many have questioned the diagnostic validity of the depression label, and raised concerns about what is seen as the widespread over-prescription of antidepressants in primary care settings (Spitzer 2007, Whooley 2010). Social scientists have explored the social, cultural, economic, political and gendered contexts in which emotional distress occurs (Ehrenberg 2010, Kokanovic et al. 2012, Fullagar and O'Brien 2012, Lafrance 2009). Further, investigations into personal accounts of emotions suggest that many people view distress as part of everyday life and its challenges, usually best addressed by mobilising personal and social supports rather than relying on medical help (Pilgrim 2007).

Against the backdrop of depression as a contested illness, people must negotiate disclosures about their depression diagnosis and treatment, asking themselves various questions. Do I have to tell my family and friends about my diagnosis? Do people need to know that I am taking antidepressants? What will happen if I tell my employer I have depression? Is it better to conceal my diagnosis? How will others judge me? In this chapter, we investigate how people who have been medically diagnosed with depression negotiate disclosure decisions both within and beyond the medical encounter, including to doctors, friends, family members and colleagues. We do this by critically analysing a selection of interview transcripts collected from people living with depression, locating our empirical findings within broader debates about disclosure as a performative and relational process (Butler 2005). We also explore how the interview pragmatics under which our data were produced shape emotional disclosures and disclosure accounts.

Research approach

The research study on which we draw involved 42 narrative interviews with women and men living in Australia who had been medically diagnosed with depression or were (without an explicit diagnosis) undergoing antidepressant treatment. Participants were recruited through mental health support organisations, snowball sampling and medical settings, including primary care and allied health. Most participants were interviewed at home. Interviews lasted from one to four hours, with most two hours in length. The interviews were conducted as part of a larger project in which personal experiences of depression and recovery were collected to develop a health information website (http://www.healthtalkonline.org/mental_health/Experiences_of_depression_and_recovery_in_Australia). All interviewees understood their stories were going to be made available, either anonymously or publicly, to a potentially mass international audience on the internet. Most participants gave permission for their interviews to be video recorded and made available online via the website, although some requested that only the anonymous audio and written transcript versions of their accounts be uploaded, or withdrew permission altogether.

In what follows, we draw on Judith Butler's essay 'Giving an account of oneself' and subsequent work this essay has inspired (Buchbinder 2010) to explore how our participants' accounts of disclosing their emotional distress are shaped by the discursive and relational dynamics in which the accounting occurs. For Butler, the self is fundamentally relational and only emerges through a 'scene of address' in which one attempts to account for oneself to a 'you', whether real or imagined (2005: 38). The scene of address is always tactical and persuasive, as the speaker seeks to recruit and act upon the listener, attempting to convince the other of the truth of their self-account (ibid.: 63). Further, the scene of address in which the self attempts to give an account is always profoundly constrained by what the 'discourse cannot allow into speakability' (ibid.: 121). Thus, any attempt to tell the truth about oneself is limited by language and social convention, as well as the relational aspects that structure all personal narratives. Which particular narrative threads will be highlighted, and which downplayed, depends on the dynamics at play in the scene of address.

Butler's work makes ethical relations pivotal to understanding narrative accounts by showing how self-accounting is both deeply relational and deeply embedded within moral frameworks. Butler derives the phrase 'giving an account of oneself' from Nietzsche (Buchbinder 2010: 115), whom she says argued that we are forced to give an account of ourselves within a system of justice. For Nietzsche, one is only required to self-account in response to an accusation. Unlike Nietzsche, Butler ultimately eschews a judicial stance towards ethics. However, by showing how self-accounting occurs within a moral framework, Butler's work draws attention to how subjects seek to position themselves according to a particular moral stance within a given scene of address. Mara Buchbinder (2010) has developed Butler's work to analyse the dynamics of research interviews as a key scene of address that shapes the kinds of self-accounts that are produced with regard to health and illness experiences. Buchbinder argues that medical institutions, like legal ones, can serve as key instruments of justice. Thus, the clinical encounter between a patient and a health professional can be viewed within a judicial framework in which patients are required to give an account of themselves and be judged according to norms of health and illness. Buchbinder (2010: 115) further argues that research interviews about health and illness can also be viewed within a 'retributive framework', insofar as such interviews index a 'crucial clinical tie' by recruiting participants on the basis of diagnosis or connection to a medical institution. In this sense, both the clinical encounter and the context of the research interview have important consequences on the ways in which research participants narrate their illness experiences and disclosure decisions. As Buchbinder puts it, Butler's work calls for 'close analytic attention to both the propositional content of narrative and the rhetorical scene in which it is deployed' (ibid.: 115).

The ideas developed in the work of Butler and Buchbinder allow us to understand that the way the subject experiences reality and gives an account of that experience is already structured by the subject's relationship to culture, language and moral frameworks. Butler's and Buchbinder's works also inspire us to investigate how the dynamics underpinning the scene of address in which disclosure acts occur – including the research interview, the clinical encounter, and personal relationships – have important consequences for how participants narrate their experiences and disclose (or conceal) their distress, diagnosis and drug treatment.

Our analysis is threefold. First, we explore how participation in our research study is itself an act of disclosure, as people are invited to give an account of their emotions, diagnosis and disclosure decisions. We explore how the disclosures and disclosure accounts produced are shaped by the context and dynamics of the research interview itself, including how participants were recruited to the study and how research questions were formulated and posed (see also Manderson et al. 2006). Second, we analyse our participants accounts of disclosing their emotional distress to practitioners in the medical context, exploring the subjectivities performed by those who disclose to medical practitioners and are diagnosed with depression. Third, we investigate the nuanced ways in which participants account for their disclosure decisions beyond the medical encounter in the interpersonal scene of address, to friends, family, colleagues and members of their broader social networks. As argued by Davis and Flowers (this volume), we suggest that for our participants, disclosing a diagnosis of or treatment for depression is not a clear-cut case of revealing medical facts about oneself; it is rather a performative and relational process, whereby people position themselves strategically in order to persuade listeners of their moral worth.

Interview dynamics and disclosure

Over the last two decades, personal accounts of illness experiences, or 'illness narratives', have become an increasingly popular subject for analysis across various disciplines. In these fields, conducting narrative interviews into people's illness experiences is now commonplace. Yet, as Charles Briggs (2007: 551) argues, scholars conducting and analysing these interviews have rarely focused sustained attention on how interviewing practices produce particular subject positions, discourses, regimes of truth and forms of authority. Briggs calls for more attention to how the complex pragmatics of interview practices – such as research proposals, recruitment practices and question guides – produce particular discourses and subject positions (ibid.: 566). In keeping with Briggs's ideas, Buchbinder demonstrates how the anthropological research interviews she conducts into chronic pain experiences form a 'curious sort of extension of the medical encounter in which patients may treat physicians – or the medical establishment more broadly – as indirect addressees' (2010: 123). Buchbinder explores how the pragmatic context of the research interview – including recruitment via medical diagnosis – led her participants to foreground headaches as the primary source of their distress, rather than complex personal autobiographies, which included experiences of entrenched social disadvantage, family disintegration and economic hardship. Similarly, in this section, we investigate how our participants foreground depression as the primary cause of their distress and position their medical diagnosis with depression as the key subject for their disclosure decisions, despite narrating difficult life stories marred by extenuating social, economic and interpersonal problems. We do this in order to explore how the scene of address in which one accounts for his or her distress – namely, the research interview – shapes the disclosure accounts produced. We focus on John's interview transcript, analysing both the content of his narrative and the pragmatic and rhetorical context in which it was produced.

John is 40 years old, married with three children, working part-time as a mental health educator. He spends the rest of his time at home caring for his school-aged children. He is well-educated and articulate, speaking calmly and eloquently about his experiences from his comfortable home. John was diagnosed with depression at the age of 37, when under immense pressure in his demanding job as a church pastor. As the size, budget and complexity of John's job expanded, he found it increasingly difficult to keep on top of things, at both work and home: 'I was working way too long, I was working way too many hours and um, I could never leave work . . . Whenever I was at home, I was kind of still mentally at work, and that created a lot of conflict between me and my wife.' John started having difficulty sleeping and became trapped in circular thoughts. At this time, his relationship with his wife deteriorated to the point where they would go days without speaking to each other. John's symptoms bore the markers of a classic depression diagnosis – insomnia, fatigue, persistent negative thoughts, irritability, difficulty concentrating and suicidal intentions. Although he was initially reluctant to disclose his problems to anyone, including his family doctor, John eventually sought medical help after he took a weekend away by himself with the intention of ending his own life. He wanted to make it appear accidental so that his children would not grow up 'thinking their dad had checked out on them', but could not figure out a way to do so. After a few days, he returned home, and self-diagnosed with depression after looking up various symptom checklists on the internet.

Even after concluding that he was depressed, John says it took him a long time to overcome feelings of shame and fear to seek medical help. John describes himself as a highly driven, results-oriented, 'Type A' person. He spent most of his childhood on a farm, but moved to the city at the age of 10 when his parents separated. The separation and move made him feel vulnerable and isolated, and he dealt with this by achieving high academic and sports results. John believes he carried this tendency towards overachieving into his adult life as a way of dealing with feelings of insecurity, and thinks it has contributed to his depression. When John eventually disclosed his distress to his family doctor, he was prescribed antidepressants. John found this difficult: 'I just couldn't take pills . . . because to me that was like the weakest thing in the world.' Nevertheless he began to take antidepressants in 'an act of desperation', because his relationship with his wife had deteriorated so badly. According to John, the medication had an immediate and positive impact on his mood. His family doctor referred him to a psychologist and, through counselling, John decided he needed to change his career. He took leave and became a stay-at-home father, allowing his wife to return to work. John then began working part-time, educating young people about depression. He embraced a biomedical view of emotional distress, endorsed antidepressant treatment and counselling, and promoted the personal and social virtues of disclosure. He was regretful that he came close to suiciding, and felt passionate about educating others about the dangers of depression when left untreated:

> I just think there are so many people out there who are suffering, who don't get diagnosed. I think it's half of all people don't get diagnosed and treated and I just think that's just like living in hell. And so I just do everything I possibly can to help get the message out there about mental health and wellbeing.

For John, promoting awareness of the dangers of depression through personal disclosure is crucial to prevent suicide and suffering.

In many respects, there are quite obvious reasons why John's narrative focuses on depression, rather than family and career circumstances, as the primary driver of his distress. Participants were recruited to this study on the basis of having a medical diagnosis of depression or because they were being treated with antidepressants, and therefore they may have assumed that the researchers were most interested in hearing about their experiences with depression. Further, many participants were informed about the study through their family doctors, or through their involvement with various different support services assisting people experiencing depression. In his role as mental health educator for a large NGO, John had ample experience in accounting for his emotional distress according to the medical narrative espoused by his employer's funding body, which frames depression as a neurochemical illness that can be fully overcome only through medical treatment. Moreover, the interview guide used in the second half of interviews encouraged participants to talk about their experiences of living with depression, diagnosis and disclosure to produce rich personal stories for inclusion on the website. Therefore, the interview pragmatics of our study – including recruitment practices and interview question guides – inevitably shaped the kinds of narratives produced.

Buchbinder (2010: 123) argues that the formal, structural dynamics of research interviews transform life stories into a 'stylised type of account', which sits in contrast to the more casual, meandering life stories produced in everyday interaction. According to Buchbinder, the context of the formal research interview about illness experience 'mandates a particular performance of self', whereby the interviewee must depict him or herself as deserving of medical care and, also, as morally accountable. John's account of his experience of depression and disclosure decisions invites his listeners – including the researcher, and the wider internet audience – to view his character favourably. John positions himself as a reluctant yet informed patient, who deserves medical care and the privileges that entails. By framing his distress as a diagnosable, treatable illness, John safeguards his right to access medical treatment, including drug treatment and counselling. He also exonerates himself from responsibility for not being able to fulfil his roles as worker and breadwinner by inscribing his decision to stop paid employment as morally responsible in that it supported his wife's ambition to return to work. Similarly, he legitimates his use of antidepressant medication primarily in terms of saving his marriage. John also positions himself as a 'mental health crusader', framing his decision to broadcast his diagnosis as a means to help others through their suffering and to prevent suicide, thus portraying himself as empathetic and morally responsible. Assuming John's life contains multiple 'narrative threads', as all lives do, by narrating his story as one of illness, diagnosis and medical treatment, John places some narrative threads at the forefront of his account while pushing others to the back (Buchbinder 2010: 123). Hence the dynamics of the research interview – including recruitment practices and the formulation of interview questions – contributed to shaping John's account towards a medicalised narrative of his experiences. We do not wish to imply that the context for John's narrative makes his story inauthentic, but rather to highlight how giving an account of oneself is always a strategic and selective process. As researchers, we need to address how the institutional structures and relations in which our interviews are conducted shape the accounts produced. Keeping interview pragmatics in mind, we now turn our attention to how the dynamics of clinical encounters between our participants and their health professionals – including family doctors, psychiatrists, psychologists and other health workers – shape the kind of emotional disclosures made in these settings.

Double disclosures and the clinical context

In this section, we analyse our participant's accounts of disclosing their emotional distress to their doctors, exploring how and with what effects emotional disclosures are performed in the clinical context. We approach our participants' accounts of their disclosures to their health practitioners as an example of 'double disclosure' (Root, this volume). Our participants' first act of disclosure to the researcher was made on the basis of their recruitment to the study, which required participants to have a medical diagnosis of depression or be taking antidepressants. By asking our participants to describe how they disclosed their emotions to their doctors, we were in effect asking them to give an account of how they disclosed. Thus, there are multiple dynamics at play in these double disclosures, including the doctor/patient dynamic, the researcher/interviewee dynamic, and the relation between the participant's past and present experiences as they recollected and reflected on their previous clinical encounters. We explore how these dynamics shape the kinds of disclosure accounts produced in our participants' narratives via an analysis of Sara's story.

Sara is 55 years old, single with no children, working as a part-time counsellor at a large university, providing support to students with mental health problems. Sara described her depression as 'melancholic depression' with a 'marked biological component'. She said she felt worse in the mornings than later in the day, had little energy for physical activity, struggled to make decisions, and found it difficult to concentrate. She described her life as being difficult from around 5 years old, when her father was first diagnosed with a degenerative neurological disease. Sara felt angry and powerless as she witnessed her father's physical and mental degeneration, followed by his painful death. Adding to her grief was the knowledge that she and her brother had a one-in-two chance of developing the same disease later in life. Sara's brother took a genetic test to determine whether he had a genetic predisposition for the disease, which came back positive; he subsequently developed the disease and died a few years before the interview took place. For many years, Sara elected not to find out her own genetic predisposition, because she was too traumatised by her father's death and her brother's illness. Sara's fears impacted upon her major life decisions including a decision to remain single and not have children. Eventually, she had the genetic test, which came back negative but, for most of her life, she believed she might have the disease. Sara's discovery later in life that she was not genetically predisposed to the family illness was a relief, but also compounded her distress because by that point it was too late for her to have children.

Sara believed she has been depressed for most of her life, but was not diagnosed until the age of 43. She recalled a combination of difficult events in her personal and working life during this period, which prompted her to consult her family doctor for a physical health complaint. She could not recall exactly how she disclosed her emotions to her family doctor initially, but said she probably did not need to say much as her physical appearance would have expressed her distress: 'They just needed to look at me [laughs] and realise that um, you know, I was very, I was very, um I was tearful, I was very um irritable, I was unable to, to do my normal daily activities. I was unable to work.'

Sara's description of her embodied pain demonstrates how emotional disclosure can be an embodied rather than verbal performance. Body language, tears, facial expressions and a generally upset demeanour can communicate emotional distress. While Sara's disclosure to her family doctor began with a physical performance, it was quickly translated into medical discourse by her doctor, who diagnosed her with depression, prescribed antidepressants, and referred Sara to a psychiatrist for counselling.

Sara recalled feeling terrified about disclosing her feelings to a psychiatrist, especially having to discuss the emotional impacts of witnessing her father's illness and death. Despite her early fears, however, at the time of the interview, Sara had been seeing the same psychiatrist for over ten years, with whom she had developed a strong rapport. She said her psychiatrist listened to her in a way that nobody else ever had done. Sara conceptualised her relationship with her psychiatrist as a strong and equal partnership, but also said there were occasions when the relationship was strained:

> She [psychiatrist] has inordinate patience, I think [laughs]. Um, she doesn't always have it right. It, it feels very much like it's been a journey that we've done together. Um, I think she has, she has a very good capacity to listen and to understand and she knows my story now . . . There aren't very many people who know the whole story. So there's something that's very important as the, her as the repository of the story, of the narrative . . . But it was also a relationship that was fractured on many occasions . . . Usually because I was being really [laughs] um well look, I think often I was being quite terrified. And I was just unable to do, to do the things that needed to probably happen at that time.

Sara's emotions became clearer to her through the act of disclosing to her psychiatrist in the therapeutic situation. Sara experienced the act of disclosing her emotions to her psychiatrist as a shared journey, in which they both negotiated the narrative that most usefully accounted for Sara's distress.

Drawing on lectures given by Michel Foucault and published after his death as *Fearless Speech* (2001), Butler argues that telling the truth about one's self always comes at a cost: 'The price of telling is the suspension of a critical relation to the truth regime in which one lives' (2005: 131). Thus, Sara's disclosures to her psychiatrist could be framed as a form of self-subjection, whereby she was required to give up a critical stance towards psychiatric power. However, telling one's story in the clinical context does not necessarily mean submitting uncritically to medical authority. Sara's conceptualisation of her relationship with her psychiatrist as a partnership emphasises the negotiation at play in their combined efforts to tell the 'whole story' of her pain. Butler argues that the basis for ethical work is not a fixed, permanent self-identity, but rather the continual desire and attempt to not close down the task of narrative itself. Thus, Sara's disclosure to her psychiatrist over a ten-year period might be interpreted as strenuous ethical work on the part of both Sara and her psychiatrist, as they sought to make Sara's experiences less opaque. Indeed, through psychotherapy, Sara gained experience in accounting for her emotions in a way that enabled her to be more open in her disclosures to friends, family members and colleagues. Although being intensely secretive about her emotions during her youth, Sara said that she was increasingly comfortable in disclosing her experiences to a small, trustworthy group of friends and colleagues. She emphasised the value of these relationships in her life, as her friends helped her to 'monitor her emotional stability', pointing out when her emotional state appeared to be deteriorating. Sara also mentioned how disclosure of her diagnosis to sympathetic colleagues had allowed her a high level of leniency and flexibility in her working life, which had been very valuable at difficult stages of her illness. Despite Sara's increasing openness about her distress following therapy, however, she was still highly selective in her disclosure decisions, as exemplified by her withdrawal of permission to use the audio recorded transcript of her interview on the website due to confidentiality concerns.

Sara's account demonstrates that disclosing emotional distress to medical professionals needs to be understood as a complex social exchange, with ramifications beyond the clinical context. Sara was unable to conceal the physical manifestations of her distress such as her tears and irritability, reminding us that emotional disclosures are inherently relational and embodied. The mere presence of another person – in Sara's case, her family doctor – can force unintentional disclosures as others observe and interpret our behaviours and appearance and relay these back to us in words. Further, Sara's description of her long-term relationship with a trusted psychiatrist shows how the dynamics of the therapeutic scene of address shape the emotional disclosures made and the stories we narrate of our lives. This is not to say that medical discourse determined Sara's self-accounting. Rather, Sara's story is one of co-authorship with her psychiatrist. Sara's disclosures in the therapeutic context also impacted on her disclosure decisions in the interpersonal sphere, highlighting the inherently relational aspects of disclosure. We examine this in the following section.

Disclosure and the interpersonal scene of address

Here, we explore how participants described disclosing their depression diagnosis or treatment with antidepressants to friends, family members and colleagues. We suggest that participants disclose in strategic, relationally tailored ways in an effort to maintain their moral standing in the face of their contested diagnosis. Recently, sociological researchers have argued that people need a witness to validate their therapeutic journey, whether this witness is a therapist, close friend, parent or colleague (Silva 2012). For example, in analysing how young, working-class people draw on the therapeutic model to narrate their journey to adulthood in an era when traditional rites of passage such as financial independence, marriage and parenthood are no longer achievable, Silva found that her research participants needed a witness to validate their newfound adult status, without which they could not fully perceive themselves as adults (2012: 519). In different ways, both John and Sara found witnesses for their distress. They accepted their distress was a biomedical problem, and the therapeutic model gave a certain pattern to their disclosure decisions. John's decision to widely broadcast his diagnosis of depression was closely linked to his belief that depression is a serious, life-threatening illness. Sara's gradual journey towards talking about her distress with others, enabled by her long-term relationship with her therapist, led her to disclose her diagnosis to family, friends and colleagues, strategically and selectively. In this section, we focus on Amelia, whose story is quite different.

Despite taking antidepressants for over fifteen years, Amelia had never formally received a diagnosis of depression. Her uncertainty about the medical legitimacy of her drug treatment, coupled with her strong resistance to emotional disclosures to doctors, friends or colleagues, meant she struggled to find a witness to validate her experiences, leaving her suspended in a narrative of suffering and isolation.

Amelia was 51 years old at the time of the interview, married, with two adult children, working as an academic at a large university. She began her story with recollections of the emotional turmoil she experienced while studying as an undergraduate student at university. At that time, she had many caring responsibilities for her mother, father and grandfather, all of whom were chronically ill. She said she felt emotionally distressed through most of her twenties, but was unable to talk to anyone about her emotions, especially her parents whom she felt she had to protect. After the birth of her first child, Amelia's emotional state worsened. She became a mother while enrolled in a PhD, and she felt that both her studies and role as a mother were compromised. Adding to her distress was the strong sense of loneliness and isolation she felt as a stay-at-home mother. She did not have other mothers to talk to about her experiences, and she felt emotionally estranged from her husband. She recalled that during this period, she did not intentionally conceal her feelings from others but, rather, felt utterly unable to talk about her emotions:

> I remember, um, hearing about places like family care centres where you could go with your baby and they would help you and all of that. And I desperately wanted to go and get some help because I was, um, not coping with looking after the baby and, um – but whenever I tried to tell somebody I really needed help [sniffs] I was so overwhelmed I couldn't say it. I felt like I really just wanted to beg for help, but I couldn't [sniffs] I couldn't quite manage to do it, because saying it made it worse kind of thing.

Amelia's recollections of her early experiences with prolonged emotional distress as a teenager and then as a young mother focus on her inability to disclose her feelings to anyone, and how the loneliness of experiencing these emotions in isolation compounded her distress. Her inability to find a confidant with whom to disclose her distress left Amelia suspended in a narrative of suffering and loneliness, which, as we discuss below, continued throughout her life as she actively concealed her distress from most people.

Despite the emotional suffering she experienced after her first child was born, Amelia consented to her husband's wish for a second child. This time, her experience was significantly better. She returned to her academic career only four months after delivery, which she felt had some emotional benefits in that she could escape from the difficulties of motherhood through her work. However, again, Amelia felt divided between her roles as mother and worker and felt unable to do either well. She continued to be unable to talk about her distress to anyone, instead distracting herself by reading novels and concentrating on her work.

When her children were in late primary school, Amelia's husband told her he wanted to leave the marriage. Amelia rapidly descended into what she describes as a 'deep depression'. Her husband later revealed that he had been having an affair with another woman, but, at first, he said only that he wanted to leave, which Amelia experienced as very frightening: 'That was just really scary for me because I just thought, here's this person who knows me best in the whole world and who lives with me, and for no reason he just wants to not live with me anymore [laughs], you know.' In the end, Amelia's husband did not leave her but, during this period, Amelia started to have uncontrollable thoughts of injuring herself. These disturbing thoughts prompted her to visit her family doctor, who prescribed anti-depressants, which she has been taking ever since, for approximately fifteen years. Despite years of drug treatment and ongoing emotional distress, Amelia did not recall ever being formally diagnosed with depression and described her encounters with her family doctor as restricted to renewing her prescription for antidepressants.

Amelia attributed her emotional distress exclusively to biological causes, namely, her hormones. She described always having severe mood changes associated with her menstrual cycle, including irritability followed by exhaustion and guilt. Amelia said antidepressants are the most helpful treatment for her depression, and she was emphatically resistant to counselling or any type of talking therapy, which she believed would be ineffective at treating her 'hormonal depression'. She also expressed fear that counselling would open up too many painful issues for her to confront, such as problems in her marriage and what she describes as 'immature parts of her personality'. She expressed fear at being harshly judged by health professionals, recounting a time when she chatted to a psychologist at a dinner party, and he described his female clients with depression as 'whinging women'. This encounter left a lasting impression on Amelia, and she returned to it several times throughout the interview:

> I think probably every counsellor secretly thinks that, you know, every woman who goes is just a complaining, whingeing bitch, and that's all I am. And just that terrible feeling that, you know, God, what right have I got to complain or whinge or feel depressed, you know? What an incredibly privileged life I have; how wonderful a life I've got. How many people out there that have got real problems? How dare I [cries] you know, take up anybody's time or resources to try and help me.

By giving such weight to this encounter, Amelia censors herself and denies the possibility that she has a legitimate need for therapeutic help. She forecloses all opportunities to fully disclose her distress in a medical or therapeutic setting, closing down opportunities to attain a witness to validate her experiences.

Further cementing her isolation, Amelia described being extremely selective in disclosing her distress and antidepressant usage to her social networks, and was particularly secretive in her work place. She had disclosed her antidepressant usage to her husband and sons who, according to her, tried to be supportive but 'do not fully understand' the extent of her distress. She was extremely reluctant to disclose her distress and drug treatment to her work colleagues, as she worried they would judge her as being incompetent and unfit for promotion. However, after years of taking antidepressant medications, she had disclosed to a small group of family and friends:

> There are very few colleagues and friends I've told – [friend's name], um, and one other friend. I got really upset one day and I felt I needed to explain to her why. Er, friends – this – there's a friend I mentioned to you. I ah, somehow or other we both let each other know that, um, we were on medication for depression. I've got two cousins [sniffs] and [laughs] I can really clearly remember, um, we went – my cousin, who lives here, um, in [city name] - we went to visit the other cousin, who lives in another city and [sniffs]. And um, the other cousin, um, was saying look, you know, I've got something to tell you girls. I've just – I've started to take medication for depression. And we just both went aaah, so do we! [screams and laughs]. It was so funny [laughs]. Oh, that was really amazing. So yes, that's – a small number of people. But I would – I feel really genuinely afraid of other people knowing because, um, I've got a really strong sense that it would diminish me in their eyes, you know; that they would not think I was as professionally competent or, you know, I, I assume that I'm right on the edge anyway, in terms of their image of me.

Being prescribed antidepressants for distress appeared to have increased Amelia's capacity for talking to carefully selected others about her distress, at least to the extent that she had reciprocated her cousins' disclosure by sharing with them her own antidepressant usage. However, disclosure decisions remained restricted by her concerns about maintaining face in her professional and personal relationships. Even with health professionals, Amelia is guarded and secretive: her encounters with the family doctor were restricted to renewing her prescription for antidepressant medication, and she had rejected numerous referrals to a counsellor. She admitted that she was nervous about participating in the research interview, as she was afraid that talking about her feelings would make her distress worse. Concealment of her distress was a personal strategy to control her relationships by attempting to avoid disapproval and negative opinions, but left her suspended in a narrative of distress.

Disclosure as a complex social performance

In this chapter, we have argued that disclosing emotional distress is a complex social performance, to be analysed with regard to the scene of address in which the disclosing occurs. We have examined three scenes of address – the research interview, the clinical encounter and the interpersonal sphere – to investigate how people disclose and conceal their emotional distress, depression diagnosis and antidepressant treatment to doctors, friends, family members and colleagues. The dynamics of the research interview – including recruitment practices and the formulation of interview questions – shaped our participants' accounts in various ways, leading them to give formal, stylised accounts of their distress and disclosure decisions. Supporting the findings of other research (Briggs 2007, Buchbinder 2010, Manderson et al. 2006), our analysis reminds us of the importance of attending to the context in which self-accounting occurs in order to understand disclosures and disclosure decisions. As the popularity of narrative interviews continues to grow within the social sciences, it is critical that researchers consider thoughtfully how the social relations underpinning their data impact on the kinds of accounts produced. We need to investigate the ways in which accounts of lived experiences are mediated through social relations, including the context of research interviews.

We have also argued that disclosing emotional distress to medical professionals needs to be understood as a complex social exchange. Dominant mental health campaigns tend to conceptualise the barriers to emotional disclosure and medical help seeking in terms of a lack of public awareness of mental illness. These campaigns focus on educating the general public about depressive symptoms to address what is framed as under-diagnosis. However, our analysis revealed that people who are aware of biomedical explanations for distress nonetheless remain reluctant to disclose their distress to doctors. People described unintentional disclosures in the clinical context as they consulted their medical practitioners for other, physical complaints, but were unable to conceal their embodied distress. For those people who decided to disclose their emotions to a trusted counsellor over many sessions, emotional disclosures were not a clear-cut act of revealing fixed self-truths, but rather a relational, discursive negotiation between doctor and patient. Further, disclosures within the medical scene of address impacted on disclosures beyond the clinical encounter, as in the case of Sara.

Personal, social, work and family contexts also impact on decisions to disclose or conceal a diagnosis of depression, with lived effects on people's sense of self and relationships. People were strategic and selective when talking of their experiences, based on personal judgements about the potential consequences for their sense of self-worth and relationships. These judgements were shaped in part by people's relation to their medical diagnosis. For those who embraced biomedical explanations for their distress, disclosure decisions took on a predictable pattern and language. Leonard and Ellen (2008) have argued in relation to living with HIV that some illness narratives are more widely available, readily produced and easily heard than others, due to the social and historical processes that privilege certain forms of knowledge. They suggest that narratives that are entered into the 'archive' can be readily accessed and used, while others 'fall out' of the narrative record (Leonard and Ellen 2008: 39). Yet for those who did not accept or felt uncertain about the medical basis of their distress, disclosure decisions were problematic. This was the case for Amelia, who failed to attain a witness for her distress.

In addition, new relationships are produced as a result of disclosure decisions. John, for instance, creates a new image of himself, post-disclosure, as a more enlightened, well-balanced individual. He sheds his former, over-achieving self in favour of what he sees as a new and improved self, more connected to his family and less career-driven. John's new identity is steeped in medical and public health discourse on depression, treatment and prevention. It has real lived effects in terms of a new career and new family responsibilities. For Sara, disclosing her depression is a means to improve her capacity for self-knowledge, self-understanding and transformation, through better monitoring of her moods. By receiving acceptance and feedback from others, Sara achieves greater self-acceptance, helping her, as she says, to make better life decisions. For others like Amelia, who choose not to disclose their emotional distress and antidepressant use beyond a very close circle of people, the lived effects of concealment are evident in descriptions of diminished relationships and missed opportunities. Amelia's intimacy with her husband is affected by her reluctance to talk about her distress, and her perception of his unwillingness or inability to listen and comprehend her emotional distress. Unlike Sara, who finds talking to others difficult but empowering, Amelia appears to find talking about depression threatening and, in some situations, impossible. Disclosing a diagnosis of depression therefore emerges as a highly strategic, partial and selective social exchange, whereby people attempt to gain social support and understanding while ensuring their character and moral worth are protected.

Acknowledgements

We wish to thank all our participants for generously sharing their experiences with us. We also wish to thank Lenore Smith for her assistance in collecting interviews, and Mark Davis and Lenore Manderson for their helpful comments on earlier drafts of this chapter. The research on which this chapter draws was supported by an Australian Research Council Linkage Grant (LP 0990229).

5 HIV/STI prevention technologies and 'strategic (in)visibilities'

Mark Davis and Paul Flowers

Disclosure is a central, but often taken-for-granted, aspect of the social interventions that seek to prevent and moderate the impact of HIV and sexually transmitted infections (STIs). Such disclosures matter in intimate life, too, influencing as they do matters of safer sex, establishing relationships and procreation. In both public health systems and in intimate life, however, there is some evidence that disclosure is coming to be articulated in novel ways with, and through, technology. Such technologies include rapid HIV test and treat interventions, social media used to establish sexual connections and enhance contact tracing for HIV and STIs, and home testing that, to some extent, bypasses traditional clinical services and their structured disclosures, as occurs with pre- and post-test counselling. These transformations have implications for the practice of sexual health and ramifications for how to conceptualise disclosure as social practice.

HIV/STI-related disclosure is commonly taken to be the communication of knowledge regarding a person's health status, their propensity for illness, or risk to others. Disclosure can be voluntary or required, done by the person diagnosed or by others, or even presumed by others. Disclosure figures in the clinic when the doctor or nurse enquires of one's sexual practices as part of risk assessment and diagnosis. Whether or not the patient discloses can shape the clinical encounter and related health outcomes. Disclosure also shades into the difficult arena of public health law which requires notification of HIV and some STIs, and the related practice of contact tracing and partner notification where patients are required to inform their sexual partners so that they can also be tested for infections and, if needed, treated. When one person tells another of their infection or disease, they influence how others see them and how their social relations will proceed, sometimes with unintended consequences. For HIV in particular, but also for other chronic STIs such as herpes, interventions seeking to reduce the effects of stigma have focused on whether to and/or how to disclose (Adam et al. 2011). Here, there is a focus on assisting people to reflect on the social implications of telling others of their status, including partners, spouses, children, family, workmates and so on (Green and Sobo 2000).

Much research on disclosure among those affected by HIV and STIs, however, relies on psychological frameworks such as 'consequence theory' (Eustace and Ilagan 2010, Kalichman et al. 2003, Mayfield Arnold et al. 2008, Serovich et al. 2008) and 'disease progression theory' (Emlet 2008, Eustace and Ilagan 2010, Serovich 2001, Serovich et al. 2008). Consequence theory is based on notions of risk and calculative reason, which imply that individuals weigh up the pros and cons of the decision to disclose to others. Factors that appear to influence such disclosure decisions include: fear of social and sexual rejection by others (Eustace and Ilagan 2010, Race 2010, Serovich et al. 2008, Sowell et al. 2003); fear of violence (Serovich et al. 2008); desire to protect others from worry (Serovich et al. 2008); gossip and violation of confidentiality (Mayfield Arnold et al. 2008, Race 2010); and concerns of impact on offspring (Eustace and Ilagan 2010). Disease progression theory assumes that individuals are forced to disclose to others when they need to access services and to manage their illness, for example, to take time away from employment. As illness progresses and becomes more physically apparent, individuals may find that disclosure becomes relatively automatic.

In response to the idiopathic inflection of consequence and disease progression theories, some researchers have conceptualised disclosure as a sociocultural phenomenon and therefore shaped by historical context, identity politics and norms. For example, researchers have established accounts of the particular ways in which disclosure is enacted in African communities, where being open about serostatus can attract discrimination, exclusion and violence (Bond 2010, Squire 2007); the social mores and moral standards that exist in gay male sexual networks (Adam 2005, Davis 2008, Flowers and Frankis 2000); and the challenges for heterosexually active people living with HIV who find themselves having to explain their serostatus to social and sexual partners who have little knowledge of HIV and the various means of its acquisition (Persson and Richards 2008).

These psychosocial and contextual accounts point to the pronounced intersubjective aspects of disclosure and its resonances for self and social experience more generally. The communication of meaning regarding oneself is axiomatic to social life. Names and other identity signs, biographical detail, experiences, intentions, emotions and desires, to name a few, can be offered to others as the means for establishing oneself as a social being, to form connections and take collective action. Such telling of oneself can be thought of in terms of the dramaturgical metaphor (Goffman 1959, 1983, 1986 [1963]) and Mead's phenomenological psychology of 'I and me' (Mead 1913), among other frameworks. The dramaturgical perspective, in particular, is a very common way of thinking about telling and disclosure, as self-presentation, both in everyday life and in social inquiry. Mead's social psychology draws attention to the dialogical relation between self-perception and self as mediated by how others are perceived to know of the self, suggesting some of the subjective complexities involved in telling. Dramaturgy and Mead's social psychology are limited, however. Among their problems, they suppose selfhood that precedes interactional life, giving us a somewhat mechanistic conceptualisation of sociality dependent on the (untenable) seminal agency of the individual.

Telling, however, can also be framed in terms of the Foucauldian elaboration of confession and care of the self (Foucault 1978, 1982, 1988, 1990). In this view, telling is a form of self-subjection: the internalisation of forms of power linked with the disciplinary carceral. Telling also mobilises pastoral power in the sense that taking up the position of teller is the means by which subjects come to consider themselves as able to tell of the self. Telling is, therefore, not simply a mediation of facts and psychic phenomena pertaining to the individual. Selfhood comes into being through the circulation, positioning, interpretation and negotiation of signs. Such performative telling necessarily relies on both 'teller' and 'audience', even if this relation is only imagined. The importance of the teller-audience relation draws telling close to narrative practices that also give emphasis to the circuits of narration and consumption in social life, as explored in other chapters in this volume.

In this chapter, we adopt the view that disclosure is complexly performative. As we discuss, this has particular salience for the pharmaceutical and social media technologies becoming important to the prevention of HIV and STIs. The disclosure/performativity/technology nexus does not simply mediate knowledge of HIV and STI status, nor is it a straightforward vehicle for the extension of biomedical forms of expertise and authority over the sexual and intimate lives of affected individuals and communities. On the contrary, performative, technologised disclosure appears to be opened up to intersubjective, collaborative and localised negotiations and strategies with a consequent proliferation of the forms that HIV and STI visibility can take.

In the following, we first consider the 'technosexual' imaginary that frames the diagnostic, pharmaceutical and social media technologies becoming important for HIV/STI prevention. We then reflect on the questions of power, self-identity and social relations implied by the use of these technologies, with particular reference to the collaborative and performative dimensions of telling and the relevance of these perspectives for conceptualising disclosure's particular expressions in connection with the prevention of HIV/STIs. Last, we explore the nuanced ways in which disclosure produces HIV and STI visibilities and effects in sexual life, by contrasting personal accounts with online sexual health interventions addressing disclosure. We draw on data from qualitative research projects conducted in the UK: one on the impact of antiretrovirals in the sexual lives of gay men with HIV (Davis 2008, Davis 2007, Davis et al. 2002); and the other concerning the e-dating practices of HIV positive, HIV negative and untested gay men (Davis et al. 2006a, Davis et al. 2006b).

HIV/STI prevention's technological imaginary

The gathering importance of technology in HIV and STI prevention reflects the more general growing importance of biotechnologies in health. These developments are associated with the changing social and economic conditions that prevail mainly in the global North, and the related expansion of scientific and technological knowledge and expectations of what biomedicine can do for health. The second half of the twentieth century was marked by the rise of surveillance medicine in affluent countries (Armstrong 1995, Lupton 2000, Petersen and Lupton 1996). This reflected an intensification of administrative interest in the management of health outcomes for populations, in part through the expansion of health surveys, the monitoring of morbidity and mortality, and the development of health education and health promotion. Over this period, affluence and public health interventions have increased the lifespans of most people in countries of the global North, accompanied by the greater burden of increasingly differentiated chronic disease (Aronowitz 2009). In addition, more diseases and disease states are being discovered, and existing diseases redefined and reimagined, together with the expansion of biomedicine's capacity to intervene (Webster 2007). In particular, new knowledge of genetics and the proliferation of information technology are increasing treatment options, enlarging patient expectations (Webster 2007), and giving rise to so-called personalised medicine. *Experimentalman.com* reports on biomedical developments in the area of personalised medicine. The website is a useful example of the dramatic changes taking place in biomedical knowhow and also of the 'possessive individualism' (Blackman 2010: 3) with which it appears to coexist. Health budgets are also expected to grow. For example, in Australia, it is estimated that expenditure will increase 189% over the period from 2003 to 2033, from $85 billion to $246 billion (Goss 2008). To contain expenditure, mitigate expectation, and pursue improved health goals, governments have increasingly resorted to technologies and the related notion of the 'expert patient' (Webster 2007). For example, online health advice services are now provided by the state in Australia (*healthdirect.org.au*) and the UK (*nhsdirect.nhs.uk*) and by private insurers such as Medibank Private (*medibank.com.au*) and BUPA (*bupa.co.uk*). These services are designed to ease pressure on outpatient and accident and emergency services. Patients accessing these sites are expected to collaborate in forms of online triage, preliminary diagnosis, and sorting out major health threats from minor self-manageable conditions. Also managing pressure in clinical services and activating self-management, in the UK during the 2009 outbreak of pandemic influenza, public health authorities implemented an online service for accessing diagnosis and prescriptions of antivirals (BBC News 2009). This approach had the additional benefit of inhibiting social contact linked with the transmission of influenza viruses.

Commerce has also entered the field of technologised, consumer-led health care. For example, GlaxoSmithKline funds *healthcoach4me.com*, a website which provides advice for the management of one's health, including stress management, weight management, diabetes and heart disease. The website simulates the coaching or counselling that one might access in face-to-face services through interactive, online technology that permits the development of personalised health goal setting. Such advice portals have proliferated, as illustrated by sites such as *doctorspring.com* in the USA and *betterhealth.vic.gov.au* in Australia. Direct to consumer marketing of genetic testing is offered by several companies (see *lumigenix.com* and *genetrackaustralia.com*) and has led health authorities to offer warnings and guidance (National Health and Medical Research Council 2008). Mobile technologies such as phones and laptops are being used to collect biological data from patients (Cleland et al. 2007) and to conduct interventions for health promotion (Lefebvre 2009).

If and when realised, the flows of biological data from individuals, through their mobile telephones and related paraphernalia, into public health systems and back again, may perfect surveillance medicine, enhancing the panoptic forms of discipline implied. Online initiatives that publish illness narratives (see *healthtalkonline.org*) can likewise be seen to be part of this transition to mediated bio-communities. Interestingly, the rapid rate of technological development (of both hardware and software) exempts much of the application of such technologies from the usual scrutiny of evidence-based medicine. By the time multi-site trials have been resourced, the technologies are obsolete, superseded by more innovative approaches. All these developments indicate the rising importance and rapidly evolving effects of the biotechnologisation of social worlds, ramifications for biosociality and, in particular, new forms and functions of health-related disclosure.

In parallel with these developments for health in general, diagnostic, pharmaceutical and online media technologies are becoming prominent in sexual health and particularly the prevention of HIV/STIs. New and intensive forms of pharmaceutical interventions are being advocated not only to treat infections but also to prevent onward transmission, for example in the form of Treatment as Prevention (TasP) and Pre-Exposure Prophylaxis (PrEP). TasP concerns prescribing anti-retrovirals for people with diagnosed infection to inhibit the chance of them infecting sexual partners, but prior to manifestation of HIV-related disease. In 2012, an international consortium of HIV experts released a Consensus Statement on the use of PrEP for HIV prevention, that is, a course of anti-HIV drugs to inhibit infection (International Association of Physicians in AIDS Care 2012). The statement implies that PrEP should be made available to those at risk of HIV infection on an episodic or semi-permanent basis. The antivirals that are normally used to treat HIV infection are now used for prevention. The idea that those who do not need them should take antivirals is novel and signifies a new mentality of the biotechnological management of HIV prevention, a shift that, as with previous milestones in HIV, is likely to come to influence the prevention of STIs in general. While much of the rhetoric of the legislative changes supporting these pharmaceutical approaches to prevention stresses that they should be seen only to complement condom use, it is possible that they will be presumed to be and so used as an alternative to condoms. This approach in turn will transform the significance and meaning of HIV disclosure (for example, HIV negative men on PrEP may well disclose this status with sexual partners).

The internet is now replete with resources, interactive forums and e-mail lists that allow people to share information and advice regarding all manner of sexual health concerns. Pfizer's *viagra.com* invites consumers to diagnose their own erectile dysfunction and to seek out prescription. In discussion forums for Viagra, participants share stories regarding their experiences – a very public although relatively anonymous form of disclosure – and circulate strategies for accessing and using the product, in some instances bypassing the prescribing physician entirely (Fox and Ward 2006). Online, personalised risk-assessment robots exist for such problems as HIV risk (see *hivaidsresource.org/hiv-testing/hiv-risk-assessment*). HIV self-testing – which operates with the same logic as pregnancy self-testing technology – is now being advocated, implying that anyone should be able to determine their HIV serostatus without attending a clinic (Frith 2007). These examples suggest that sexual health care is now not restricted to the confines of a fixed, bounded clinical setting: it is increasingly networked and dispersed in the media-scapes of astute and willing consumers. Moreover, the boundedness of the state in matters of sexual health provision and jurisdiction is questioned. For example, it is possible to import HIV self-testing kits from countries where they are legal (e.g. the USA) to countries where they are not (e.g. the UK).

The disclosure of HIV and STI status figures in these developments, either indirectly, as in the example of PrEP, or more explicitly in a variety of online interventions. Public health practitioners in the USA have used emails to conduct contact tracing among gay men who may have been exposed to syphilis (Adams 2004). Gay men use the internet to find sex partners but, in many instances, the names and contact details of these partners are not known. Such lack of information means that these men cannot be contacted in the usual way by letter or telephone. Public health practitioners have resorted to using online dating email systems to contact men and ask them to have tests for syphilis (Klausner et al. 2000). Public health practitioners have also proposed that e-dating websites should include sexual health descriptor fields in online profiles so that e-daters can indicate their health status, including, for instance, 'date of last STD screening, HIV serostatus, and genital herpes or genital wart history' (Levine and Klausner 2005: 55). Some consumers already disclose some aspects of their health in an informal manner (Davis et al. 2006a, Davis et al. 2006b, Race 2010) and some e-dating websites enable users, if they so choose, to make statements regarding their sexual health and intentions regarding safer sex and condom use. Online chat between potential e-daters on these topics is also regular (Davis et al. 2006a, Davis et al. 2006b, Race 2010).

These developments are not necessarily associated with improvements in sexual health. While user-driven forms of e-pharmacy enable the sharing of treatment stories and access to cheap, generic forms of erectile dysfunction drugs, physicians worry that such e-pharmacy bypasses their expertise, leading to misdiagnosis and untreated side-effects. The expansion of 'sexuo-pharmacy' raises the spectre of commerce-driven medicalisation of sexual health (Conrad and Leiter 2004). Indeed, the search for the 'pink viagra' – sexual dysfunction treatments for women – occupies drug companies interested in expanding their lucrative sexuo-pharmacy market (Hartley 2006). The aesthetics of the penis are open to increasing commodification and commercial exploitation (Flowers et al. in press). In addition, over the period when sexual health technologies have taken form, rates of sexually transmitted infections have inclined steeply. Arguably social media have created radical new sociosexual spaces and opportunities for sexual mixing outside the normative cultures of heterosexuality (see, for example, *plentymore-fish.com/uk_dating/*). Reported diagnoses of chlamydia in Australia have doubled in the period 2001–11 (Kirby Institute 2011). New HIV infections have also trended upwards in this period, with an 8.2% increase between 2010 and 2011 (Kirby Institute 2012). These developments indicate that the increased use of technology may weaken – and not improve as intended – sexual health outcomes.

There are additional problems. The empirical basis for assessing the benefits and drawbacks of sexual health technologies is patchy, with substantial gaps for sexually transmitted infections, including HIV (Imrie et al. 2007). It is not clear, for instance, how newer technologies articulate with the established technologies of sexual health. Moreover, as mentioned above, there are inherent problems with constructing an evidence base on such a rapidly changing terrain. There is no systematic account of the extent to which social media refashion or even displace the counselling and pedagogical technologies that were hitherto the mainstay of sexual health interventions outside the confines of diagnosis and treatment. The proliferation of technological approaches to sexual health also raises questions for how sexual health, and indeed sexuality, will come to be defined and practised in contemporary life. For instance, it is unclear if sexual health technologies re-assert 'absence of disease' models of sexual health and, if they do, how they articulate or not with rights-based models, which define sexual health in terms of the 'rights of all persons to have the knowledge and opportunity to pursue a safe and pleasurable sexual life' (World Health Organization 2010: iv). The ways in which sexual health technologies mobilise absence of disease and rights-based models are flashpoints for the definition and practice of sexual health in the twenty-first century.

These new technologies do not only have practical effects in the lives of those affected by HIV/STIs, nor do they only create opportunities and dilemmas for the public health professionals concerned. They suggest also the mobilisation of what it is imagined technologies can do for the prevention of HIV/STIs, in particular, and for sexual health more generally: what could be called a 'technosexual' imaginary of what might become possible. Codes of conduct for the online communication of STI and HIV status are key examples of this imaginary since they imply that, through the manipulation of self-representation, the prevention of HIV and STIs will be furthered. It is anticipated that public health rationality of disease control will therefore be extended. Other important examples of this technosexual imaginary, however, come from the online bricolage of consumers outside of those technologies run and advocated by public health systems. For example, websites such as *herpes.com* direct people with the infection to dating sites where they can meet other people with the same status, thereby allowing people to avoid or delay having to disclose their status. Similarly, people with HIV use websites to establish like-with-like sexual contacts, where disclosure of infection status is redundant. Gay men's barebacking websites work with a similar logic, combined with an explicit eroticisation of such practices (Davis 2009). Researchers have investigated the extent to which 'serosorting' via websites occurs in groups affected by HIV (Butler and Smith 2007, Mao et al. 2006). Such like-with-like organisation of sexual contact depends on some forms of disclosure of HIV and STIs status, explicitly or otherwise. The technosexual imaginary, therefore, frames both public health systems' approaches and the creatively, transgressive bricolage of consumers. It is productive of multiple approaches to, and configurations of, the prevention and amelioration of HIV and STIs and related practices of disclosure.

Technosexual imaginary, self-identity and the impossibility of full disclosure

The imaginary giving form to HIV/STI prevention technologies has implications for self and interpersonal life that go beyond those already discussed. As noted, disclosure is performative of intersubjective experience. Disclosures construct identities and relations with others. They are also collaborative in the sense that there is always a discloser and a disclosee, imagined or otherwise.

The disclosures particular to HIV and STIs mean that biomedical knowledge is implicated in such intersubjective relations. Biomedical signs such as 'HIV positive' and 'HIV negative' or others like these – necessary for the communicative enactment of HIV and STI disclosures – are implicated in the imaginary of what technology can do for sexual health. Indeed, the particular ways in which online forums can fix and circulate biomedical signs lie at the heart of the technosexual imaginary: that is, as if such communication assures action to prevent the transmission of HIV and STIs that face-to-face and verbal communication does not. It would be possible, then, to argue that disclosing knowledge of HIV serostatus, for example, is a reflection of biomedical power and therefore the incorporation of subjects into systems of medical labelling, authority and imperative. At least for HIV, however, biomedical power does not necessarily operate in this way. In particular, identity talk and disclosures in relation to HIV reveal productive and creative biopolitical action on the part of those affected by HIV. Such biopolitical action takes account of the interpretive possibilities and challenges of the use of biomedical signs and the always partial, contextual ways in which disclosures are enacted.

'I am HIV' is used, not exclusively but with impressive regularity, in spoken discourse, and was discernible in interviews done in London with gay men with HIV in relation to the impact of antivirals in their lives (Davis 2008, Davis 2007). We could take such identity talk to be an example of medicalisation: the labelling of self in medical terms or a kind of making over of identity according to the language of viruses (Flowers and Davis 2012). However, closer attention to such identity talk suggests something different. Identity talk brings medical knowledge and self-subjectification close together, but not simply as a matter of constraint. In particular, 'I am HIV' can be understood as metonym and synecdoche. 'I am HIV' is short for 'I am HIV positive'. But it can also be interpreted, metonymically, as self-talk where HIV is associated with the self and is taken on as an identity sign. Synecdoche goes one step further, to suggest that HIV is recognised as a *part* of the self and therefore stands for the whole self.

To illustrate, consider Edgar's reflections on sex with his HIV negative partner and HIV transmission:

> I don't know or whether he sort of believes enough in his mind that we will always be together so it wouldn't really matter if he becomes HIV anyway 'coz he wants to share that with me. I don't know. I don't know whether he thinks in his heart that he loves me so much that if he became HIV, it wouldn't really matter to him you know . . .
> [and later]
> Him becoming HIV through me.

'Becoming HIV' has the double metaphorical quality of 'I am HIV'. HIV works by integrating itself into host cells. These cells are used to produce more HIV ultimately destroying the host cell. In this view 'becoming HIV' synecdochally summarises a complex biological process within the body. However, we know also that HIV diagnosis is a social process of identity formation. 'Becoming HIV' is then also metonymic for a loose connection between HIV infection and self-identity, an effect of social relations rather than corporeal. This double metaphor of self with HIV complicates, even troubles, how we want to think about biomedical power and identity and, relatedly, how disclosure with regard to HIV at least, is practised. In a variation of this self-applied metaphorical language of HIV biomedicine, Edgar comments:

> Yeah coz we discussed this the first time I saw you that whole bareback riding thing
> Yeah . . .
> You know it's such a big chance to take that you could be well like I've been and then get, you know, shagged by another virus and then become really quite ill you know coz that virus could be completely different to the one you've got which you probably would be coz they all are anyway more or less aren't they . . .

Edgar speaks of being 'shagged by another virus' to describe the situation of reinfection, where the HIV positive person can be infected by a virus of another genotype that is resistant to HIV treatment. This language is tongue-in-cheek but, like 'I am HIV' and 'becoming HIV', it summarises a complex process of biological and social transformation. Reinfection and the genotyping of HIV are examples of medicine's new hi-tech approach to disease. Edgar is engaging with these new technologies and applying them to matters of sexuality and identity.

The point here is that identity talk informed by biomedical knowledge is not a simple matter. A somewhat habitual but playful use of metaphor can be used to make various connections between self and biomedical knowledge and its new proliferating technologies. These language games suggest the operation of medical power in identity and lifeworlds, but not simply as top-down subjectification. Metaphor enables as much as it constrains, mobilising discursive practices, making it possible to speak of the new complexities of HIV technologies and the biological and social changes implied. Such metaphors also have the effect of multiplying selves: a self as the biomedical HIV object; a self as manipulated through treatment; self as a risk to others; and a narrating/observing self. They represent a kind of appropriation of biomedicine or, in other terms, an engagement with innovations in biological and social effects and the meanings connected with them. They suggest that the imaginary space for what technology can do in sexual worlds embraces the creative engagements with questions of self and relations with others. Diagnostic categories and related biomedical knowledge regarding infection and treatment can be used to lay claim to identities under transformation and manipulation. These practices suggest a looser, more mobilising, hybridising, even playful, co-constitution of biomedical signs and self. They indicate an opening up of possibilities rather than a closing down, or at least a negotiation of the terms by which biomedical power shall rule. This makes sense, too, since, as discussed, health care is in a period of rapid transformation under new scientific insights, technological possibilities and economic imperatives.

Biomedical signs of identity implicated in disclosure, however, are not simply or only transferred: they are subject to collaborative hermeneutics where signs are mutually accepted, but also subject to creative recontextualisation and reinterpretation to give them new connotations and effects. This perspective also opens up disclosure to the possibilities of misinterpretation, ignorance and resistance, capturing more ably the indeterminate and ambiguous aspects of social life. Following Judith Butler's line of argument in *Giving an account of oneself*, insolubly partial telling – partial because of what is forgotten, repressed, unknown – conditions social life and poses the practical and ethical challenges of whether or not and how to collaborate in the quest for meaningful social existence. As Butler puts it:

> My account of myself is partial, haunted by that for which I can devise no definitive story. I cannot explain exactly why I have emerged in this way, and my efforts at narrative reconstruction are always undergoing revision. There is that in me and of me for which I can give no account. But does this mean that I am not, in the moral sense, accountable for who I am and for what I do? If I find that, despite my best efforts, a certain opacity persists and I cannot make myself fully accountable to you, is this ethical failure? ... Is there in this affirmation of partial transparency a possibility for acknowledging a relationality that binds me more deeply to language and to you than I previously knew?
>
> (Butler 2005: 40)

Telling of oneself then joins the teller and their interlocutor in a social project for the establishment of the self-other relation, and the meanings that make that possible. Butler also suggests that:

1) The relation of self to oneself may not be wholly transparent. Aspects of self can remain untold and important events and relations escape telling. Material and embodied presence too may remain non-narrativisible, but nevertheless significant to lived experience.
2) One cannot author the conditions that make one's story intelligible to others. Norms, conventions, expectations condition when and how stories get to be told.
3) One's story depends on the 'structure of address' that makes it possible. Social settings such as a conversation, a research interview, biographical writing, an online blog, among others, shape also how stories are made.

Understanding the act of telling of oneself as performative yet partial and constituted in specific circumstances with particular effects on self and relations with others provides a novel way of conceptualising disclosure in connection with the prevention of HIV/STIs. In particular, subjects are required to take on HIV/STI disclosure and to consider its implications for self and related norms and expectations, as Edgar's account suggests.

Subjects are compelled to consider the structures of address that constitute HIV/STI disclosure, such as the clinic, intimate life or other relevant contexts. Disclosers and disclosees are joined together in these identity-related expectations and practical considerations. But, perhaps most importantly, HIV/STI disclosure binds all in consideration of its potential failure. According to Butler, such failure need not be reason for despair, but is actually the 'real work' of disclosure.

A useful illustration of the interpretive challenge of disclosure comes from a print-based advertisement from a 2000 campaign conducted by the Terrence Higgins Trust in the UK. The advertisement features a blurred image of two men in a near embrace and the text: 'Assume nothing: It's your shout. No one mentioned condoms.' 'I assumed he must have HIV too.' 'I assumed he was HIV negative like me.'

The advertisement tells a story, telegraphically, of a sexual encounter where condoms were presumably not discussed and therefore not used, a practice mistakenly rationalised in two ways. The HIV positive subject assumes that the sexual partner, by not requesting condoms, is also HIV positive. The HIV negative subject makes the same 'he-must-be-like-me' assumption, with the same effect on condom use. The particular example addresses the misalignment of assumptions regarding seroidentity in the sexual encounter. It therefore addresses non-disclosure, that is, the situation where the absence of biomedical signs (as opposed to the verbal utterance of them) connotes HIV identities in ways that can lead to (false) assumptions of serostatus which can contribute to the risk of HIV transmission. The advertisement is designed to serve as a warning of such misinterpretation or 'failed' disclosure. It is therefore an intervention into the practical/ethical ambiguities of disclosure in sexual contexts. It demonstrates the difficult terrain traversed by HIV education in the context of the circulation or not, as the case may be, of biomedical signs that help to make the prevention of HIV possible. The advertisement also reveals an interest in how people affected by HIV manage biomedical knowledge of themselves and others, a focus that is, arguably, now central to the newly technologised forms of HIV/STI prevention. As approaches that focus upon biotechnological prevention blossom, the ambiguities and complexities of associated possible disclosures will also multiply. The disclosures, and/or their absences, wrought by both PrEP and TasP, for instance, trouble the simplistic and traditional dichotomy of HIV status. New subjects reliant upon biomedicine to avoid HIV will be both positive and negative and new questions will emerge concerning self, identity and disclosure.

Strategic (in)visibilities

Self-identity talk reflects imaginative deliberation: where metaphor and notions like 'shagging viruses' make it possible to speak of self-identity and sexual practice in novel ways, both reflecting technological possibilities that arise in biomedicine, and opening up biomedical knowledge and effects to creative and productive uses. The ever-present partial quality of disclosure implicates already metaphorical and multiple biomedical signs, such as 'HIV positive' and 'HIV negative', in the hermeneutics of escaped meaning and related implications for interactional life. As noted in the discussion of the technologies being used to support the prevention of HIV and STIs, disclosure can be done by denotation or by context, that is, by using biomedical signs in online communication or by choosing social contexts where disclosure is redundant. As will become clear, the nuances and complexities of the disclosure–performativity–technology nexus exercise questions of biopolitical visibility, with some surprising turnings in the methods and effects of HIV/STI disclosure, including de-articulation from some of its social ramifications, or so it would appear.

For someone with HIV, presenting one's diagnostic status online can have a markedly dual quality of benefit and drawback. In this extract, Gavin reflects on his experiences of disclosing HIV serostatus in e-dating chatrooms:

> [Y]ou get people that come into a room and harass people 'cos they've got HIV. You get a lot of that. Even the ordinary chatrooms like in the London chatroom you'll get, you know, there's a couple of people who are obviously disturbed ... you get messages come up in the main chatroom, not personal to you, but they'll say 'fuck off you AIDS b***' and all this sort of thing or 'this person's got AIDS' or 'keep away from him' and things like this, you get all of that sort of thing there so you put yourself up for that when you go in there ... some people just look at the pictures and say 'oh you look a bit thin in the face' then as far as they're concerned you know you've got AIDS and that's it. But you know, yeah I was really harassed a lot last year by this particular guy and every time I went into a chatroom he would start on me ...
>
> (Davis et al. 2006b: 168)

Gavin's account underlines how online HIV disclosures can attract prejudice, perhaps in ways that are more flagrant than in offline social interaction. Experiences such as these raise questions of how online communication constitutes social interaction. Some analysts argue that it is the relative anonymity of online communication in chatrooms – where visual cues are not present – that leads some people to transgress social norms (Ben-Ze'ev 2004, Cooper and Griffin-Shelley 2002, Ross et al. 2006, Whitty and Carr 2006). Such views subscribe to technological determinism, however, overlooking how transgression is possible in other interactional contexts and the complex ways in which online communication can be applied to the moderation of social effects. For example, in other accounts of their experiences with chatrooms and disclosure, gay men with HIV talk of using online technologies to test out if potential sex partners might have prejudices (Davis et al. 2006b). Disclosure is thus employed to pre-empt the chance of embarrassing or distressing face-to-face social interaction. Chatroom technology and newer modes of relating facilitated by app-based technologies, much like identity-talk under new HIV technology, already discussed, offer their own possibilities for disclosure.

In the following example from an online chat-based interview, David makes it clear that the new media can be put to work to figure disclosure as negotiation of sexuality, desire and community:

David: I set up a new profile that said 'Never' to safe sex and I was completely blatant about my HIV status – it was only alluded to in the former profile . . .

David: I had changed my old profile to use some of the euphemisms to allude to POZ status so I presume he did . . .

MD: what are some of the euphemisms . . .

David: 'Positive outlook on life' . . .

David: My uncompromising stance is less than 12 months old.

David: Yes.

MD: What uncompromising stance is that?

David: That I only have unprotected sex.

MD: What made u change?

David: Realising that I much preferred it.

MD: What made u adjust yr profile?

David: For the majority of the period since I was diagnosed I had had only protected sex.

MD: Can u expand?

David: Realising that every man was out for the most pleasure HE could get – why should I not have the same rule?

MD: So is this a way for you to get pleasure while reducing HIV risk?

David: It is also only in the last 15–18 months that I had realised there was such a large subculture of POZ men having unprotected sex.

MD: What made u realise that?

David: I think that the number of profiles on gaydar explicit about that has risen markedly in that period.

MD: How do you feel about being open about yr status on the net?

David: I think it is important.

(Davis et al. 2006b: 166–7)

Disclosure here is figured as the raison d'être of online existence. Biomedical knowledge makes an appearance incorporated into a mode of sexual engagement that is self-affirming. By implication, openness about one's status is the way into forms of sexual interaction where stigma and the risk of new HIV infections are excluded. David's practice is a form of serosorting, as noted above. It is also consistent with Edgar's account, discussed previously, where metaphorical biomedical signs were applied to the com-plexities of the biological and social transformations linked with HIV diagnosis and the effects of treatment on the risk of transmission in sexual practice. David's use of online technologies is another way of engaging with the implications of diagnosis for sexual life. Following Butler's schema, David's online disclosure reveals an engagement of self with oneself, a reflec-tive arrangement of identity signs with effects in mind for self-identity and social/sexual relations. Such disclosure also instantiates collective action in the sense of the claim on a biosocial organisation of sexual community figured around HIV serostatus. The conditions of disclosure – in this case the online chat technology – give rise to particular denotations and con-notations of biomedical identity which invite interlocutors into the practical and ethical dimensions of interpretation. Such disclosures and how they can be interpreted are collectivising, too, in the sense that they bind disclosers and disclosees together in hermeneutical action, with implications for the forms that sexual interaction can take.

Disclosure such as this can therefore be understood as onto-performative of identity and social relations. Disclosure is not subservient to immanent biomedical truth, which asserts itself at particular moments. Nor is disclosure an act of biomedicalisation in any simple way. Disclosure appears as the negotiation of volition and constraint. Such communicative enactment of negotiated biomedical power articulates into social worlds, or perhaps even, articulates social worlds into being. This account also reveals an imaginary of social existence where the implications of HIV, through this form of disclosure, are bracketed out by making HIV serostatus visible. HIV is effec-tively made invisible in social worlds, by making it visible.

Such strategic visibility is in evidence in other domains of sexual health. In 2008, the Melbourne Sexual Health Centre launched the text service *letthemknow.org.au*, which allows those diagnosed with STIs such as chlamydia, gonorrhoea and syphilis to send an anonymous SMS to sexual partners who may have been exposed to the infection. The SMS reads: 'A message from letthemknow.org.au. [Name of recipient] u may be at risk of Chlamydia. Pls have a sexual health check. See website or phone [Telephone number supplied] PLEASE DO NOT REPLY.'

The initiative is consistent with calls from public health authorities to use social media creatively to address sexually transmitted infections. It also represents responses to the rise in notifications of STIs. For example, chlamydia infections in Australia increased from 74/100,000 in 1999 to 272/100,000 in 2008. One way of reducing new infections would be to test and treat the sexual partners of diagnosed patients. This method of disease control relies, however, on patients informing their sexual partners. *Letthemknow* is designed to make such disclosure more frequent. It is straightforwardly a public health intervention into a difficult terrain justified because of the burden of disease, the growing scale of the problem and a concomitant lack of robust evidence to inform sexual health interventions.

Letthemknow is state sponsored, research driven and public health sanctioned. Though outwardly unlike David's approach to disclosure, discussed above, *letthemknow* can be understood to employ strategic visibility. For example, *letthemknow* makes reference to 'anonymous SMS', offering anonymity as a possibility for patients. In this way, patients can make the implications of their diagnosis visible to their sexual partner(s) without (in theory) exposing their identities. Anonymity, however, is called into question if the recipient of the SMS has only one partner. Only those with more than one partner will not know who sent them the message. Only in some circumstances, then, the website offers a kind of non-identified disclosure, disclosure pared down to its biomedical utility and freed of any other of its social ramifications, at least for the discloser. Even in situations where the sender of the SMS is known or is assumed, the website offers an 'at arm's length' form of disclosure. Like David's imagined technosexual order, *letthemknow* also inspires a vision of the eradication of disease through the careful orchestration of disclosure without disclosing. Like David's account, it articulates with an imagined network of sexual connection.

Conclusion

Understanding HIV/STI disclosure as performative gives purchase on the social implications of the combinations of diagnostic, pharmaceutical and social media technologies being employed in sexual health care. Disclosure's intersubjective and collaborative nature and its partial qualities draw attention to the practical and ethical ramifications of the technologies of HIV/STI prevention. To some extent, these technologies are already responses to the practical and ethical challenges of preventing HIV and STIs. But they also reveal a technosexual imaginary, where it is assumed that the careful arrangement of biomedical signs in online life will contribute to the proper management and eradication of disease. This imaginary is partly realised and partly aspirational, without much critical reflection on what kinds of technosexual citizenship that will come into being.

Speaking of one's biomedical identity, however, need not be a simple matter of taking on medicine's labels and authority. As noted, metaphorical identity talk helps to appropriate biomedicine so that its effects and imperatives are rendered multiple and negotiable. This can be true of disclosure through social media. Disclosure practices give rise to strategic visibilities that re-configure the practices of disease prevention. Identity labels, like HIV serostatus, can be made visible so as to render aspects of self-identity less visible. Disclosure can be enacted without disclosing, as in the case of *letthemknow*. Central to this technosexual imaginary is the assumption that effects in lifeworlds can be produced with the careful arrangement of biomedical signs in online life.

While the circulation of signs to make one's biomedical identity invisible and disclosures without identification may solve some health problems, they may lead to others. The two examples discussed suggest proliferation and complexity as opposed to unity and coordination. David's example seems to refer to a way of thinking about sexual health that embraces pleasure, community and volition. *Letthemknow*, of course, relies on the 'absence of disease' definition of sexual health. These competing definitions of sexual health appear to be difficult to reconcile, particularly as HIV disclosure appears to be taken on as a personalised practice with implications for sexual community, while the disclosure of chlamydia, for instance, can be de-identified. By implication, different expectations and privileges articulate with different diseases and those most affected by them. The expected proliferation of biotechnological disclosures will likely present these challenges and more. As indicated by the examples discussed in this chapter, and in other chapters of this volume, such complexity and its attendant ambiguities will be key. This challenge of ramified and partially opaque disclosures, however, need not be overwhelming. As Butler suggests, the communication of biotechnological signs which escape meaning need not set us apart: such ambiguous disclosures could bring us together in newly ethical, social forms.

6 Is it 'disclosure'?

Rethinking tellings of genetic diagnoses

Devin Flaherty, H. Mabel Preloran and Carole H. Browner

There are all kinds of secrets; there are all kinds of tellings. When patients are diagnosed with a genetic disease, a variety of different terms are used to characterise the processes involved in letting others know of their diagnosis. Our aim in this chapter is to complicate the assumption that one of these terms, 'disclosure', is an appropriate way to characterise what occurs when people tell others they are afflicted with a genetic disease.[1] While 'share', 'inform', 'reveal', 'tell' and 'communicate' are also often used to describe this particular kind of telling, most authors combine these terms and use 'disclosure'. But they are careless about the specificity of the latter term, and take it to be a simple descriptor of an act of communication (e.g. Petersen 2006, Claes et al. 2002, Ormond et al. 2003, Henneman et al. 2002, Featherstone et al. 2006, Burgess and d'Agincourt-Canning 2001, Smith et al. 2002, Lehmann et al. 2000, Forrest et al. 2003, Klitzman et al. 2007).

We problematise the assumed interchangeability of these terms. 'Disclosure' makes certain implicit claims about the teller, but these are rarely explicitly investigated. In particular, we problematise three aspects of the concept of disclosure in the context of a genetic diagnosis: first, that the person receiving such a diagnosis necessarily does so as a separate and autonomous individual; second, that the diagnosis is, for the recipient, something unwelcome and unwanted, that it is 'bad news'; and third, that the recipient is, or will be, invariably stigmatised by their genetic diagnosis. Our overarching claim is that 'disclosure', as it is generally understood, should not be assumed when analysing what takes place when people with a genetic disease tell other people of their diagnosis. Such telling must be repositioned as a particular kind of self-revelation that occurs only when certain pre-conditions are met.

To do this, we draw on the cases of fourteen individuals recently diagnosed with Huntington's disease (HD). Huntington's is a highly penetrant, autosomally dominant movement disorder, a group of diseases and syndromes that cause a person to produce movements that are too weak, too forceful, too uncoordinated or too poorly controlled for the task at hand.

In addition to Huntington's disease, the class of movement disorders includes Parkinson's disease, multiple system atrophy, the ataxias (e.g. Friedreich's ataxia, Machado–Joseph disease, spinocerebellar ataxias), essential tremor, restless leg syndrome, dystonia, stroke, cerebral palsy and encephalopathies. Personality changes and declines in mental acuity may be part of a movement disorder disease, as they are with Huntington's. Symptoms typically begin in middle age, around 40, and individuals die on average fifteen years after onset (Evers-Kiebooms et al. 2000).

The Huntington's disease cases which inform this chapter are drawn from our larger study on the meanings and uses of genetics and genetic testing information for patients suffering from progressive, degenerative movement disorder symptoms, and for their family caregivers and their clinicians (Browner and Preloran 2010). Most salient to our focus here on genetic disclosure is that our study participants had been suffering from undiagnosed movement disorder symptoms and were seeking a diagnosis or had just recently received one. Most other work on the experiences of genetic diagnosis has looked at individuals and families at risk for, but not necessarily experiencing, symptoms of a genetic disease (Hallowell 1999, Cox and McKellin 2001, Almqvist 1999, Evers-Kiebooms et al. 2000, Chapman 2005, Bloch et al. 2005, Huggins et al. 2005, Etchegary 2006, Koenig and Stockdale 2011, Burgess and d'Agincourt-Canning 2011, Konrad 2005). The arguments we put forth as to the inapplicability of 'disclosure' to people such as those in our study stem largely from the fact that they were already in the midst of illness.

Some authors, most prominently Katie Featherstone and colleagues (2006), as well as Monica Konrad (2005), have similarly sought to dismantle 'disclosure' as a default descriptor of genetic diagnosis tellings, problematising the idea that disclosure is a one-time offering of a self-contained piece of information. As Featherstone and colleagues write:

> [I]t is highly misleading to think in terms of 'information' that is shared equally and explicitly [among family members] . . . There can be no assumptions that in the everyday world family members 'share' information in an explicit fashion, if at all. It is nearer to the truth to think in terms of fragmentary disclosure, partial disclosure, or even 'family secrets'.
>
> Featherstone et al. 2006: 52

Konrad comes to similar conclusions regarding disclosure, though derived from a different theoretical perspective, describing genetic diagnostic tellings as a pragmatic kind of 'drip by drip' approach to truth telling that is sensitive to the timing of disclosure and to how knowledge is conveyed, rather than to any pure ontological sense of unmediated substance. 'An ethics of disclosure, in other words, works itself out over time as *a series of staggered revelations*' (Konrad 2005: 101, emphasis ours). For these authors, their problematisation of disclosure is largely focused on a telling as a one-time, revelatory occurrence. Konrad and Featherstone and colleagues seek to emphasise the pragmatic contexts of family life and the vicissitudes of everyday life to bring to light the idealised nature of a discrete information transfer from one family member to another. Their projects are not to question the term 'disclosure' itself, but to problematise the paradigmatic action of telling.

While we also seek to complicate the way we think (and write) about genetic diagnostic tellings, we aim not to dismantle the concept of a discrete telling itself, but to show that when describing such tellings, the use of 'disclosure' is not necessarily accurate or appropriate. Importantly, we do not here give accounts of any of the tellings of the participants in our study. Through a comparison of our participants' stories with the dominant language in the literature, we discovered that it would not be appropriate to apply 'disclosure' to their tellings. As previously mentioned, our insights stemmed largely from the fact that our participants were already suffering from movement disorder symptoms. Therefore, by virtue of their very visible physical symptoms they could not keep the fact of their condition private, even if they had wished to do so. This led us to reconsider the use of 'disclosure' as a neutral term that could be unproblematically interchanged with 'inform', 'share' or 'tell'.

Below, we examine three indexed aspects of disclosure: that people encounter their diagnosis alone as autonomous individuals; that their diagnosis is necessarily 'bad news'; and that they feel stigmatised by it. We argue that because these individuals were already sick (some for many years) when they received their diagnosis, the conventional concept of disclosure did not apply.

Research methods

As noted, the cases that we consider in this chapter were drawn from a larger study, recruited from the practices of thirteen neurologists who diagnose and treat movement disorders in a major US metropolitan area. The patients of these neurologists were invited to participate in our study if they were seeking a consultation with a new neurologist for their movement disorder symptoms, as previously defined. Because prior to the consultation there was no way of knowing whether the patient already had, would ask for, or would be offered genetic testing, all new patients who reported at least one movement disorder symptom were recruited. At the conclusion of data collection, those with no direct experience with genetic testing became part of a comparison group.

The study involved a structured observation of the initial clinical encounter between a neurologist, a patient and any accompanying individuals, followed some time later by in-depth interviews with the patient and any accompanying family members. In all, we observed 125 new patient intakes and interviewed 116 of those patients. We also opportunistically interviewed nine patients of neurologists who were not formally part of the clinician sample. Forty-seven of the seventy-one relatives (66 %) who accompanied patients agreed to be interviewed as well.

Preliminary data analysis revealed that one-quarter (n = 31) of the patients had either undergone genetic testing before entering our research project or were offered it during the course of our investigation. Of these, fourteen tested positive for Huntington's disease. In comparison with our larger sample of 125, this HD subset was younger (mean age = 48.4; larger sample = 56.0), more likely to be male (58% versus 51% in larger sample), and far more likely to be born in the USA (58% versus 39%). It is these patients and their family caregivers to whom we now turn our attention.

The patient unit

In conventional use in the biomedical field, the term 'disclosure' implies that individuals come to know their diagnosis alone and that they deal with the information independently and autonomously, before then choosing whether or not to reveal their diagnosis to others. This use of the term relies on the notion of an individual, autonomous subject. Yet the competing idea that 'the family is the patient' is integral to the practice of genetic medicine, because one patient's positive gene test indexes potential diagnoses for the patient's blood relatives as well (Etchegary 2006, Petersen 2006, Chapman 1992, Finkler 2000). The concept of autonomy has a complicated relationship with genetic diagnoses, as the diagnoses are both clinical – so subject to the privacy and confidentiality norms of any other clinical diagnosis – and are innately shared:

> Family ties can take on a new meaning in genetics and challenge our usual view of confidentiality. To whom does genetic information belong: the individual or the family? What right does one family member have to learn the genetic results of another member? What obligation do people have to tell others in the family of their own test results and inform other family members that they are at risk?
>
> (Pembrey 1996: 76[2])

Since Pembrey's chapter, these tensions have largely been discussed in terms of the decision of whether or not to get tested in order to obtain a genetic diagnosis (Smith et al. 2002, Biesecker 1998, Burgess and d'Agincourt-Canning 2011, Hallowell 2003, Burke et al. 2003). Thus, as late as 2006, Etchegary claimed that '[f]rom a clinical perspective, genetic test decisions should be autonomous and voluntary. No other person or group should unduly influence this decision' (2006: 65). Although in current medical genetic practice, and especially in genetic counselling, some professionals make efforts to include the family in decision-making processes (Forrest et al. 2003), the issue remains unresolved: 'The familial implications of genetic information can lead to a conflict between a physician's duties to maintain patient confidentiality and to inform at-risk relatives about susceptibility to genetic diseases' (Lehmann et al. 2000: 705).

A more accurate representation than an autonomous individual or an entire family is what we came to call the 'patient unit': patients (the individuals known to be carrying the genetic mutation) experienced their sickness and medical treatment *along with one or more others*. Being 'in this together' was a common refrain expressed by all patient units in our research. Not only did they embody this attitude in their daily lives, they also commonly repeated this phrase in interviews: 'We're in this together.' In this regard, knowledge of the genetic diagnosis rarely seemed to reside exclusively with a patient. We attribute this mainly to the fact that most people in our study lived with family members (generally their spouse) and were already sick: they were actively cared for by them.

For example, siblings Mary and Roland (pseudonyms) exemplified the characteristics of a patient unit. Both in their fifties, we met them at the clinic where they had come to explore treatment options for Roland's recently diagnosed Huntington's disease. Roland had been suffering from movement disorder symptoms for many years, causing him first to lose his job as a jazz musician and take up another as a taxi driver, until his rapidly declining memory forced him to leave that job as well. He was homeless for several years. When he was arrested for vagrancy, he called his estranged sister, Mary, to bail him out of jail. Since then, Mary has become Roland's devoted caregiver. Roland chose to stay at a boarding facility despite Mary's invitation to him to move in with her and her husband. While the siblings did not live together, their lives were deeply intertwined.

Roland was one of the more severely symptomatic patients in our study: his memory was extremely poor; he experienced a marked declined in his everyday mental acuity; at times he had difficulty speaking and controlling his movements. While it was necessary for Roland to have a caretaker, Mary and Roland's relationship had become extremely close, far beyond what was needed for Mary to simply tend to her brother's day-to-day needs. For instance, Mary took full responsibility for keeping detailed track of Roland's medical history (they both referred to her, jokingly, as his 'secretary'). She had an intimate knowledge of his current state of health and his past courses of treatment, and participated with Roland in joint interaction with the neurologist. Throughout the intake consultation, brother and sister shared the floor, effortlessly accomplishing the interactional dance that is the telltale sign of intimate daily familiarity. Smiling at each other, making quiet jokes, the warmth between the pair was palpable.

Mary was also instrumental in getting Roland tested for HD. As Roland recounted, 'Mary hooked it up with the test . . . the one test they wouldn't do for some reason was for HD . . . [but] I finally tested positive last month.' Mary also frequently spoke of herself as having 'had him tested'.

This obviously diverges from established models of patient autonomy and disclosure: because the severity of Roland's symptoms prohibit him from acting as an autonomous subject in the medical setting, Mary serves as his proxy decision-maker. Mary's insistence, as caregiver, that Roland get tested precluded the possibility of him disclosing his diagnosis to her. Of course, given her extensive involvement in his care, Roland was not in a position to keep his diagnosis a secret – to choose not to disclose – even if he had wanted to. For this reason we argue that for patients such as these, disclosure to their family caregivers – in the conventional biomedical sense – is precluded by the closeness of the relationship and the patient's needs for care.

Another patient unit was Edward and Sarah, an elderly married couple. They attended Edward's neurological consultation together with their two daughters and a granddaughter. All five interacted with the physician, asking questions, providing information about Edward's medical history, and articulating the family's most pressing concerns: Edward's accelerating personality changes and growing memory problems. In separate interviews, the couple spoke of jointly making decisions about Edward's diagnosis, treatment and care and, most importantly, whether he should be tested for HD. Here, Sarah describes their decision-making process: 'We came home to talk about it, because we always like to come home and talk ... I told my friend we were thinking of having the test.' Sarah's use of the plural pronoun 'we' here, also frequently used by Roland and Mary (e.g. 'we finally got the test') indexes the felt sense of togetherness that was the core, unifying characteristic of those we regarded as patient units, further problematising the meaning of disclosure in the context of genetic testing.

Tom and Teri, also a married couple, often expressed their togetherness through reference to the expediency of having two people instead of one to deal with the continual everyday issues that arose from Tom's ongoing medical care and declining health. For example, when we asked Tom why Teri had attended the neurology appointment, he said, 'She needs to know what's going on ... It helps to have two people because it helps to have that extra ... like she can write notes down.' Teri explained that she drives Tom wherever he needs to go and that it was she who had found the neurologist they were seeing: 'I had excellent referrals from other Huntington's disease patients and family members that referred me.' While the practicalities of dealing with Tom's medical care often seemed foremost for this couple, they also frequently expressed a felt sense of togetherness that went beyond mere expediency. For instance, in Tom's statement that Teri 'needs to know', he makes it clear that any clinical information about his condition must be conveyed to them both. The notion of patient autonomy inherent in 'disclosure's standard biomedical definition is irrelevant in his situation. Moreover, in Teri's characterisation of crucial medical referrals for her husband as referrals made to *her*, she explicates their shared perspective that they are 'in this together'.

The experiences of patients like these complicate the assumption that the relevant parties in the telling of a genetic diagnosis are an autonomous individual with whom the physician will disclose test results, on the one hand, and whosoever they decide to tell, on the other hand, assumptions made when such tellings are characterised in terms of the orthodox and individualised 'disclosure'. Instead, we observed allied and supportive patient units where diagnostic and related biomedical information was conjointly received and managed, in the instance of life partners supporting each other but similarly in family groups whose members have a personal stake in learning their relative's diagnosis since they, too, may have inherited the illness. These dynamics are likely not limited to our small set of patients, but rather might play a role in the experiences of many, particularly those already involved in intense caregiving relationships. These patients were not, and did not feel, alone in their daily illness, and concepts of clinical autonomy or confidentiality did not apply to them.

Not simply bad news

We next seek to question the notion that disclosing a genetic diagnosis provides information that is necessarily unwelcome or unwanted. We can understand this intuitively by attempting to use 'disclosure' to describe wanted diagnoses, such as learning you are HIV negative, discovering you are pregnant when you have been trying to have a child, or finding out that a tumour is benign. When something is 'good news', it might be 'shared' but not 'disclosed' in the sense that it is typically understood. The term disclosure, then, can be taken to index the diagnosis being told as *not good news*. Going one step further, we suggest that 'disclosure' is typically seen to index news as *bad news*.

Many studies have investigated the psychological effects and real-life experience with new-found genetic information, but the focus has been on the receipt of *predictive* information (Hallowell 1999, Hallowell et al. 2003, Konrad 2005, Cox and McKellin 1999, Almqvist et al. 1999, Chapman 2005, Bloch et al. 1992, Huggins et al. 1992, Evers-Kiebooms 2000, Meiser and Dunn 2000; for exceptions to this, see Hess et al. 2009, Browner and Preloran 2010, Featherstone et al. 2006, Claes et al. 2002). Such predictive information is, we maintain, quite different from receiving a diagnosis for a condition whose symptoms one is already experiencing. In this section, we show that some genetic diagnoses indeed offered patients and their relatives something other than 'bad news'.[3]

As might be expected, each patient arrived at their diagnosis by a different route, so the diagnoses did not hold consistent valence or meaning. We came to see that this variation was largely based on how they imagined their diagnosis fitting into their life stories and their personal illness narratives (Hunt et al. 1990, Browner and Press 1996). These meanings powerfully influenced how these patients felt about their diagnosis. To make this point, we offer two cases in which patients took their diagnosis to be vindicating, and one where the patient interpreted his diagnosis as merely a formal label for a disease he felt certain he had.

Before introducing these cases, more background is needed on how, procedurally, individuals are tested for HD. Huntington's is a fairly rare disease (its prevalence is now *c.* 12 per 100,000), and its testing is never part of any routine clinical work-up. People are tested only if at least one blood relative is known to carry the Huntington's gene or because they are manifesting symptoms consistent with the HD trajectory. But because many neurodegenerative movement disorders have similar symptoms, even presenting with symptoms characteristic of HD does not guarantee that a physician will order an HD test. Several in our study had to specifically and repeatedly request the test over a number of years as they searched for the cause of their symptoms: they were on what is commonly known as a 'diagnostic odyssey'. These experiences strongly affected what their eventual diagnosis meant to them.

For example, by the time we met Ana, a 37-year-old divorced woman with two young children, she had been seeking a diagnosis for symptoms she had been experiencing for fourteen years. After watching her father die in 1990 of what had been clinically diagnosed as HD, when the genetic test was not yet generally available, Ana struggled to get doctors to take her claims of illness seriously. Ana was certainly the least symptomatic patient in our research. She presented as completely healthy, which was part of her problem in attempting to be diagnosed. During the neurological consultation that we observed, she reported that she was experiencing memory decline and loss of concentration, had frequent and persistent leg tremors, and did not have full control of her movements. Yet, despite all of this, and despite the many doctors she had consulted, she repeatedly failed to secure an order for an HD test. This was mainly because these clinicians felt her reported symptoms were not consistent with early manifestations of HD: they attributed her somatic manifestations to anxiety or 'stress'. When the test was eventually ordered and approved by her insurance company, it was given based on family history, not symptoms.

When Ana's test came back positive, she experienced a rush of feelings, including anxiety and dread, especially about her ability to continue to care for her children. But counterbalancing these feelings, she felt deeply vindicated: 'I wanted to have [the test] because I knew that I had HD like my father, but I couldn't prove it. Nobody believed me; now that I have the test *nobody can deny it* . . . The test gives you the certainty that you are not crazy . . . You know that you have a real problem and nobody can say otherwise.'

Ana's attitude appears quite bold in contrast with, in the more conventional sense, what we might typify as 'disclosure', which presupposes that the diagnosis is not wanted and is conveyed to others tentatively or anxiously. Ana had sought her diagnosis for years, and it was proof that her experience of illness was based in reality, not in her head. Physicians, Ana's mother, her sister and ex-husband had long attributed her disquieting leg sensations and other problems to her 'highly strung' nature. When we asked her ex-husband, Robert, what it meant to him that her HD test was positive, he replied, 'Be more patient. Be more understanding. Listen to her a lot. *Now it is real.*' Robert, like Ana, felt that her HD diagnosis legitimised her experience, one invalidated for over a decade.

Susan expressed similar feelings of relief and vindication upon receiving her own HD diagnosis. Like Ana, Susan (age 54) had been searching for a diagnosis for years 'to find out what was wrong . . . I was so anxious to find out . . . I didn't care what the answer was. I wanted to know I wasn't crazy.' Susan's symptoms were much more noticeable – 'stumbling and falling a lot', constantly dropping things, and losing her memory and concentration, for all of which she felt responsible (as common among symptomatic individuals, see Hess, Preloran and Browner 2009, Meiser et al. 2005, Sankar et al. 2006). While upset by her diagnosis, she was also relieved 'because [now] I know I'm not crazy . . . there is a reason for the way I am'. Like Ana, Susan's HD diagnosis also explained her changing behaviour: her diagnosis was vindicating.

We now briefly return to Tom to demonstrate a very different way that an HD diagnosis can be sought by a patient or, in this case, a patient unit. A 47-year-old systems engineer, Tom had been experiencing movement disorder symptoms for several years. He had left his job, about a year before we met, due to significant decline in his motor abilities. Knowing his family history, he was almost certain that his symptoms were indicative of Huntington's. As they worsened, his wife, Teri, began researching the range of possible causes and came to agree with Tom that his symptoms were most likely due to HD.

Although Teri had wanted her husband to be tested about a year before he agreed to do so, Tom felt he just was not ready. In the meantime, however, the two attended HD support groups and researched possible treatments. By the time we met him, Tom had decided to get tested because, 'It was just the time in my life when I needed the answer . . . *I knew I had it*, but wanted to live a normal life for as long as I could. I waited until it got worse to get tested.' What he meant, and what he repeated frequently, was that he felt he could 'handle the answer'. Yet he also said he already 'knew' he had it, making the 'answer' more a formal confirmation than the resolution of uncertainty.

Seeking to understand the range of meanings associated with disclosure by patients like Ana, Susan and Tom led us again to question the extent to which disclosure is a universally meaningful concept for patients diagnosed with Huntington's. Ana's, Susan's and Tom's diagnoses and related tellings were made meaningful through their incorporation into life and medical narratives which framed the diagnosis, not as something that happened *to* them, but as actively sought by them. Their positive diagnosis was helpful to them in ways that a negative diagnosis could not have been, in vindicating their own experience (for Ana and Susan), relieving themselves of blame and responsibility for their changing behaviour (Susan), and confirming their beliefs about their state of health and eventual fate (Tom). These cases illustrate what surely is a more common phenomenon, demonstrating that 'disclosure' should not be simplistically applied to genetic diagnostic tellings.

Stigma

Our third aim is to question the assumption that 'disclosure' necessarily indexes the prospect of stigma. A number of studies of experiences of genetic disease, and studies of medical disclosure more generally, presume the salience of stigma to the topic (Ablon 1992, Sharpe et al. 2006, Forrest et al. 2003, Klitzman et al. 2007, Meiser et al. 2005, Kenen 1994, Chapple et al. 1995, Browner and Preloran 2010, Hess et al. 2009, Petersen 2006, Etchegary 2006); see also discussions of HIV disclosure (e.g. Flowers et al. 2006, Parker and Aggleton 2003, Herdt 2001). Yet stigma was not an important feature of our participants' experiences. In this section, we briefly offer some thoughts as to what might account for its apparent absence.

Stigma has been extensively studied by social scientists, most famously with Erving Goffman's iconic work (1963). Recent efforts at addressing the concept of stigma, with some mixture of a theoretical and ethnographic focus (Yang et al. 2007, Link and Phelan 2001, Oyserman and Swim 2002, Sayce 1998, Major and O'Brien 2005), have articulated a plethora of approaches to understanding stigma, how it makes itself known (or, for some, is created) in interaction, and its effects. While some argue that 'stigma' necessarily implies structural discrimination (Link and Phelan 2001), others hold that 'stigma' is a limiting concept that indexes only the feeling of being stigmatised (Sayce 1998). Many argue that stigma is inherently linked with relationships of power (Link and Phelan 2001, Parker and Aggleton 2003), while Yang and colleagues (2007) have argued that stigmatising the other is best understood as a pragmatic strategy to protect what is at stake in one's moral world. The intensity and deleteriousness of stigma assumed by various authors also vary, from leprosy (Opala and Boillot 1996) to step-parenthood (Coleman et al. 1996). And many have noted its varied definitions (Link and Phelan, 2001, Parker and Aggleton, 2003, Vernon, 2012) – some a far cry from Goffman's early claim that '[b]y definition, of course, we believe the person with a stigma is not quite human' (1963: 5).

Many recent contributions to stigma studies explicitly criticise Goffman's approach, particularly what has been interpreted as his individualistic focus (see Vernon 2012). However, we find Goffman's analysis of the social creation of stigma, particularly his examination of its relationship with stereotype, to be illuminating in considering the possible emergence of new stigmatising 'marks', such as genetic disease. Despite the various definitions of and approaches to stigma that have emerged in recent decades, we find the concept of stereotype to be as salient as ever to definitions of stigma.

Our argument on the lack of stigma found among participants in our research hinges on the relationship between stigma and stereotype, which we re-articulate below. Importantly, the design of our research did not allow us much insight into the structural discrimination that our participants may have faced, which prohibits us from either weighing in on the importance of structural discrimination to the concept of stigma, or contributing to the study of genetic discrimination, an important domain in its own right (e.g. Billings et al. 1992, Barclay and Markel 2007, Hudson 2007, Hudson et al. 2008, Greely 2005). Therefore we limit our discussion to the *experience* of stigmatisation or 'self-stigma' (Vernon 2012, Jones et al. 1984, Barclay and Markel 2007), sometimes also described as the effect of social stigma on self-esteem (Crocker and Garcia 2006, Quinn 2006; also see Crocker et al. 1998, Vernon 2012).

The concept of stereotype is fundamental to stigma, as Goffman noted: 'A stigma . . . is really a particular kind of relationship between attribute and stereotype . . . [s]tigma management is an offshoot of something basic in society, the stereotyping or "profiling" of our normative expectations regarding conduct and character' (1963: 61). According to Goffman, stereotyping causes stigma in two ways: individuals are stigmatised because they belong to a negatively stereotyped category (e.g. sex workers), or they are stigmatised when there is a disconnect between the stereotype of the identity they most prominently display (e.g. successful businesswoman) and the biographical realities of their lives (e.g. a successful business woman who is discovered to also be a successful sex worker). Goffman describes this as the difference between people whose characters are *discredited* and those whose characters are *discreditable*.

This notion of 'normative expectations' is key to the relationship between stereotype and stigma. They can be so constricting that, as Goffman notes half-jokingly, and in pure 1963 style, '[i]n an important sense there is only one complete unblushing male in America: a young, married, white, urban, northern, heterosexual Protestant father of college education, fully employed, of good complexion, weight, and height, and a recent record in sports' (1963: 128). Stigma is, then, a process that occurs 'wherever there are identity norms'. The question we pose in relation to our study is whether there are normative expectations for genotype. Is this notional white, urban, northern male also without genetic abnormalities?

Our contention that stigma was not a significant part of our participants' daily lives emerged not from our research focus, but rather from getting to know them, although some of our standard interview questions did open up fields of discussion where feelings of stigmatisation could have been expressed. For example, we asked:

- What fears or concerns did you have about getting genetic testing?
- Did deciding about genetic testing upset you in any way?
- What aspect of your condition is the most difficult for you to bear?

(We asked these same questions of caregivers, simply substituting the patient's name for 'you'.) While the sentiments expressed in response to these questions, and others like them, varied widely, stigma did not appear to be a primary concern.

One exception from our larger sample was a family of three siblings who had suffered since childhood with an undiagnosed progressive muscle disorder that affected their ability to walk and use their hands in a normal manner. Each of the three siblings was symptomatic to a differing degree and each one's life had been differently affected by feeling stigmatised by those around them. Pedro, the only brother, said that he was mocked and marginalised as a child in Mexico, and he had lost his one chance to marry because his girlfriend's mother did not consider him a suitable spouse for her daughter. She had said to her daughter: 'How can you think of marrying him? Don't you see he is defective?' (Browner and Preloran 2010: 70). In contrast, younger sister Maria married and raised two healthy children but she, too, endured feelings of stigmatisation. Like other study participants, Maria wished for a genetic (or any) diagnosis, in part because it would be vindicating: 'This illness is very shameful . . . If they would say to me that this sickness comes from the family in a certain form, it would be a relief. Because everyone would see once and for all that we're not lying . . . Everyone would know that . . . I'm not fooling anybody' (Browner and Preloran 2010: 71).

Two complementary arguments account for why this family's experiences were the exception to the more general pattern we observed: that felt stigma was not a significant part of patients' everyday experience or their sense of self. The first is, simply, that these patients and family caregivers had overwhelming, immediate everyday concerns far more consequential for their lives than any feelings of stigma or stigmatisation. This resonates with Flowers' and associates' study of disclosure and stigma in HIV-positive black African immigrants to the UK: for many of their study participants, being HIV positive was just one concern among many, including being separated from their partners and children, being financially destitute, and generally trying to make their way in a society that was largely hostile to them (Flowers et al. 2006: 113). For these individuals, therefore, stigma was a large part of their experience (especially with regard to their feelings about disclosure and associated anxieties about further social exclusion). This notion of competing concerns seems quite applicable to the experiences of our own study population, as is clear in the cases discussed above when getting an accurate diagnosis was a pressing, ongoing concern. Simply put, the illness experiences of patients in our study were not dominated by stigma as they had much more pressing things to worry about.

Our second, complementary, argument as to why stigma did not figure prominently in our study participants' daily lives is based in theories of the social construction of stigmatised groups. In considering stigma with regard to genetic illness, two potential sources of stigmatisation can be present: the illness itself and the genetic anomaly causing it. In some work, such as in Joan Ablon's studies of dwarfism and neurofibromatosis (1972), the distinction is simply not made (see also Shuttleworth and Kasnitz 2004). In this regard, Sankar's and colleagues' study of sickle cell anaemia, cystic fibrosis, deafness and breast cancer is informative. This study compared the experiences of people with conditions whose aetiology was genetic, with those with these same conditions whose aetiology was non-genetic. The authors conclude that felt stigma was not correlated with the disease's source, that is, there was no 'extra' stigma felt by individuals whose disease was genetically-based as compared with those whose disease was not (Sankar et al. 2006).[4] In our work, even the most severely symptomatic patients did not appear to experience an increased sense of felt stigma after receiving their genetic diagnosis. We argue that the lack of felt stigma expressed by the visibly symptomatic patients in our research is due to the lack of normative expectations regarding genotype.

Many have noted the importance of 'shared cultural knowledge' to the formation of stigmatised identities (Quinn 2006: 89, Vernon 2012, Link and Phelan 2001). Indeed, shared cultural knowledge is constitutive of the concept of stereotype. Thus, while it has become a familiar trope in studies of Western medicine that the influence of genetic science is growing, and soon will come to dominate the practice of biomedicine, general genetic awareness has not yet come to fruition: as yet, we are not socially aware of our own or others' genes, and thus there is no stereotyping based on genetic abnormalities (cf. Rabinow 1996). While there is a general awareness that certain familiar diseases have a genetic origin (e.g. Down syndrome), and negative stereotypes associated with many of them, a genetic anomaly in and of itself is currently not a socially meaningful phenomenon. Differences in genetic make-up are socially invisible. Link and Phelan capture well the importance of this distinction for the existence of stigma:

> The vast majority of human differences are ignored and are therefore socially irrelevant ... The full weight of this observation is often overlooked because once differences are identified and labeled, they are typically taken for granted as being just the way things are – there are black people and white people, blind people and sighted people, people who are handicapped and people who are not
>
> (Link and Phelan 2001: 367)

We therefore suggest this as one important reason why our study participants did not feel stigmatised and why stigma did not arise as a pressing concern for them. This complements our argument that these patients and caregivers had 'other things to worry about'. If genetic abnormalities had been more socially salient, stigma might have emerged as more consequential.

Conclusion

Our objective has been to complicate the uncritical, simplistic use of the term 'disclosure' to describe what happens when people tell others they have tested positive for a disease-causing gene. Our findings contrast with the overwhelming majority of similar research, which has focused on healthy individuals. The particularities of our population of already sick people illuminated critical aspects of their experiences that led us to question the applicability of the term 'disclosure' as it is commonly employed. First, no one in our small sample had to come to terms with their diagnosis as independent, autonomous individuals. Although here we have focused mainly on a minimal dyadic unit, it was not uncommon for a far more extensive network of family members to be intimately and extensively involved in the quest for a diagnosis and subsequent treatment and other life decisions. Second, although their diagnosis was generally unwelcome (clearly, they would much rather have been suffering from something less devastating than Huntington's disease), the diagnosis was neither surprising nor understood as 'bad news'. Third, patients did not appear to feel stigmatised by their Huntington's diagnosis.

We end by narrowing our perspective and then broadening it. Narrowly, we want to be clear that we are not claiming that 'disclosure' is never a useful or accurate description of the telling of a genetic diagnosis: we can certainly imagine instances where it would be an accurate use of the term as it has been typically employed. However the term 'disclosure' denotes certain specific characteristics about a diagnostic telling that cannot be assumed. These are empirical questions. More broadly, we suggest that our findings likely apply to other diagnoses. This again is an empirical question. But also, we have demonstrated that it matters what we call these tellings, because the way we describe them can connote profoundly powerful things about the people enacting them.

Acknowledgements

Research was supported in part by NIH grant 1 RO1 HG003228-01, Carole H. Browner, Principal Investigator and by the UCLA Center for Culture and Health. We thank the patients, family caregivers and physicians who graciously participated in our investigation, and Warren Thomson, Maria Christina Casado, Jennifer Musto and Marissa Strickland for their expert assistance.

Notes

1. While in the past this term had been limited in the medical field to describing the act by which a medical professional informs a patient of her diagnosis, many authors today use it to describe the telling of a diagnosis by the patient themselves.
2. See also Featherstone et al. 2006 and Finkler 2000 for discussions of individualism in the face of genetic knowledge.
3. Studies that have investigated the psychological impact of predictive testing for Huntington's show that pre-test psychological adjustment is the best predictor for long-term post-test adjustment (see Meiser and Dunn 2000 for a review of these studies). When predictive testing results are experienced as 'bad news', it might be at times appropriate to describe tellings of those results as 'disclosure'; this, however, is not our focus here.
4. Meiser et al. (2005) show that for individuals with bipolar disorder and their family members, a genetic aetiology for the condition was seen as *reducing* the stigma of the condition within the family, although it was perceived that a genetic aetiology would not affect the stigma of bipolar disorder in the broader community.

7 Disclosure as method, disclosure as dilemma

Matthew Wolf-Meyer

I heard of Jack during a grand rounds meeting at the Midwest Sleep Disorder Center (MSDC), where he was presented as a case to the assembled doctors, technicians and staff. Dr Richards, the senior staff neurologist, narrated the case. Jack was a white man in his mid-fifties, who had first experienced symptoms related to narcolepsy in his late thirties. At the time, he assumed that his daytime fatigue was related to stresses at work, and he would often contrive ways to sleep in his office or in his car in the parking lot. When he awoke, he often experienced hypnogogic hallucinations, and so he ensured that he never had to wake up quickly to attend to a workplace demand. He would also often wake up in the middle of the night and find it difficult to return to sleep. At first he assumed this had to do with his daytime naps, so he tried to stop napping during the day in order to consolidate his sleep at night. He found his caffeine consumption during the day quickly increasing, but this strategy did not seem to work. His most worrying complaint was his experience of cataplexy, the sudden loss of muscle tone, which caused him to lose his grip on things he was holding, or to fall down while walking. These bouts were brought on in periods of heightened emotion, usually when Jack was laughing with a colleague or friend.

In many ways, Jack's case is unexceptional for a narcoleptic. What was exceptional – and the reason why Dr Richards was presenting his case – was that Jack was a heart surgeon in the hospital that housed the MSDC, and the attending staff, comprised of physicians, research scientists, nurses and technicians, were being presented with an ethical dilemma: Should they reveal to the administration that one of the doctors on staff was a narcoleptic?

Jack had hoped the doctors at the MSDC would prescribe him medication that would alleviate his narcolepsy symptoms, but that this would be masked as medication for other syndromes. Narcolepsy, although very treatable with the current pharmaceuticals used for it – modafinil to promote alertness and Xyrem to consolidate sleep and relieve cataplexy events (Wolf-Meyer 2009) – carries a social stigma, and public knowledge that Jack was receiving this medication would place him into a high risk category for his medical malpractice insurance. The conversation that followed Dr Richards' presentation of the case was fairly charged – the physicians understood what was at stake for Jack, and sympathised with their peer. But they were equally worried about their field. What if a narcoleptic, using drugs off label, were to commit malpractice? The negative publicity would surely impact on them and they might be legally culpable. The debate reached no resolution, as was Dr Richards' intention in presenting it to the group: he considered the case as an exercise in ethical thought.

I reflect herein on the role of disclosure in ethnographic writing and the ethics that limit the possibilities of full disclosure. My interests are similar to those of Dr Richards: the use of disclosure as the basis for thinking through ethical problems. To discuss the act of disclosure from an ethnographic perspective, I present the same two cases from my research on sleep in the United States (Wolf-Meyer 2012) at increasing levels of fictionalisation. That is, taking a page from late modernist fiction,[1] I present the same two cases three times each with each presentation more fictional than the last – increasingly removed from the empirical situation I originally describe – enabling me, therefore, to disclose more about the cases. As the ethnographic cases become more fictional, I am able to disclose information that would be incriminating or troublesome if these details were presented in the more factitious versions. But, even as I foray into fiction, the presentations continue to borrow from fact, that is, the facts of the cases discussed and facts about sleep and its history in the USA.

I am interested in the tension between ethnographic verisimilitude and facticity precisely because it lies at the heart of ethnographic writing (Clifford and Marcus 1986), and exists in institutional tension – between social scientists and their institutional review boards, between researchers and their informants (Brettell 1996), and between writers and readers (Iser 1978). Thus, part of my intent here is to think through the act of disclosure in ethnographic writing as a methodological concern. Secondly, and this is the motivation for my interest in these discursive acts of disclosure, in this chapter, I attend to the institutional and material consequences of disclosure. For both Jack and Ryan, whose experiences I discuss below, the consequences of their disclosures endanger their status as employees and, by extension, their ability to meet their family obligations and other social commitments. Their differential abilities to disclose their conditions in their workplaces impact on my own ability to discuss their cases, as information of their cases could lead to the possibility that co-workers, family members and social acquaintances might identify them beyond their pseudonyms, leading to workplace difficulties. This might be unlikely – we all write on the assumption that a lay reader is unlikely to come across this chapter and follow the cases, and to make inferences about the individuals they know – but the shadow of this possibility limits my ability to make ethnographic disclosures, precisely because it may have material consequences for the individuals involved. Central to modern institutional review board (IRB) and human subjects guidelines in the United States, like ethics committees elsewhere, is the

assumption that the disclosure of the health status of individuals –
particularly regarding disability – may have employment consequences and
unintended social ramifications for the depicted individual if readers can work
through the data to discern the individual's identity, however unlikely that
may be. Nonetheless, modern ethnography has accepted this risk, leading to
the slightly fictionalised forms that ethnographic writing is now marked by.
I am interested here in the ethics of ethnographic disclosures – what might
be said and what may not be – and the constellations of knowledge that this
produces (Faubion 2011).

These problems of representation in ethnographic writing have been
continuing concerns in anthropology from the 1970s (Hymes 1974) and
particularly the 1980s, when critical attention to social science claims of
objectivity resulted in a move towards reflexivity regarding the situated
knowledge production of the ethnographer (Clifford and Marcus 1986). The
most lasting impact of Clifford's and Marcus's critiques of ethnographic
writing in *Writing Culture* (1986) may be the conventions that ethnographic writers now incorporate into their writing to make their work more
'novelistic'. That is, rather than the presentation of demarcated social realms
(e.g. Evans-Pritchard's discussion (1940) of Nuer religion, kinship, political oecology, etc., as properly isolated from one another), contemporary
ethnographers are more likely to integrate these social forms into discussions
of events, life histories and everyday action – usually associated with a theme
identified by the author (for three very different cases, see Biehl 2005,
Bourgois and Schonberg 2009, Das 2006). One might conceptualise this
mode as relying more extensively on the disclosure of the ethnographer about
what he or she claims to know and less upon acts of disclosure on the part
of his or her informants about their experiences, which may trouble the
veracity of the ethnographic text, but is necessary if ethnography is serving
as a mechanism of social critique (Marcus and Fischer 1986). Ethnographers
are now resolutely part of their texts (see, for example, Helmreich 2009,
Martin 2007): this might be taken as evidence that the critique of objectivity
lodged by Clifford and Marcus, and their collaborators in *Writing Culture*,
has profoundly changed the art of ethnography and its aims. Central to these
changes, I argue, is the place of doubt in the production and interpretation
of ethnographic texts; this doubt is rooted in the performance of social
scientific authority on the part of authors and the interpretive strategies of
readers, both of which depend upon the understanding of acts as disclosure,
fictionalisation and concealment as integral to ethnography.

These concerns about representation, subjectivity, fiction and truth are
indebted to trends within literary and cultural studies, now quite far
removed; however, it is worth returning to Eric Auerbach's discussion of
mimesis in literary writing (2003 [1953]). For Auerbach, modernist writing,
which social science writing is surely part of, is indebted to the 'realism' he
attributes to biblical writing, as divergent from the 'rhetorical' writing
associated with legend. Auerbach characterises realist writing with these

qualities: 'Certain parts brought into high relief, others are left obscure, abrupt, suggesting influence of the unexpressed, "background" quality, multiplicity of meanings and the need for interpretation, universal-historical claims, development of the concept of the historically becoming, and preoccupation with the problematic' (Auerbach 2003 [1953]: 23), which might also be read as an apt description of contemporary ethnographic writing. Leaving aside the relationship between Christianity and contemporary social science (Cannell 2005), the struggle for verisimilitude on the part of ethnographic writing is intended to both convince the reader of the author's experience, as well as those experiences of others that the author is representing to the reader. The basis for the author's argument and, by extension, the basis for critique, is founded on a scientific, mostly objective understanding of the conditions being reported, however contrived or bracketed these conditions are (Haraway 1997, Shapin and Schaffer 1989).

But what if ethnographic writing hewed more closely to the rhetorical, the discursive production of fiction? Auerbach describes the quality of rhetorical literature in the following way: as a 'fully externalized description, uniform illustration, uninterrupted connection, free expression, all events in the foreground, displaying unmistakable meanings, few elements of historical development and of psychological perspective' (Auerbach 2003 [1953]: 23). While some contemporary ethnographic writers employ some of these tactics, very few social scientists use all of them: this self-imposed limitation is based upon the author's desires to be seen as making scientifically sound claims (see, for example, Taussig 1997). However, the rhetorical opens up a number of possibilities for the presentation of ethnographic data, not least among them the ability of estranging the reader. For Darko Suvin (1979), and later Fredric Jameson (1991), realism is important precisely because it can be subverted; the power of most science fiction and 'postmodern' literature is that it is first able to convince its reader of the reality being described, and then is able to subtly – and sometimes radically – unsettle the reader's conceptualisation of reality. By doing so, the reader's reality becomes destabilised and the applicability of the text – its interpretive latitude – becomes greatly expanded. Like ethnographic writing, acts of disclosure often traffic in the language of the real. They must appear 'real' or based in truth in order to be full disclosures. But might more rhetorical disclosures ('I have a friend with a problem . . .') produce similar or even more profound effects, both for the discloser and his or her audience?

Knowingly skirting the conceits of realism allows me to momentarily present my ethnographic bona fides. From January 2003 through April 2007, I conducted archival and ethnographic research, first in the Twin Cities in Minnesota, and then in Chicago, Illinois. The research began at the pseudonymously named Midwest Sleep Disorder Center (MSDC), where I would attend weekly case discussion meetings and departmental lunches, as well as visit the overnight sleep clinic. I conducted formal and informal interviews with clinicians, researchers, patients and their families at the clinic and throughout the Twin Cities. At the same time, I attended local support groups for individuals diagnosed with obstructive sleep apnea and restless legs syndrome, and conducted archival research at the Wagensteen Historical Library of Biology and Medicine, housed at the University of Minnesota, and containing medical monographs from the nineteenth and twentieth centuries. In February 2006, I relocated to Chicago to conduct further research: archival research at the Special Collections Research Center at the University of Chicago's Regenstein Library, and ethnographic research with patient support groups throughout the Chicago Metro region. Coextensive with these two in-depth field research periods, I attended local and national professional meetings for sleep physicians and researchers, as well as national support group meetings for less common sleep disorders, especially narcolepsy. Over these three-and-a-half years of research, I informally interviewed more than eighty disordered sleepers, and conducted life history interviews with an additional forty. In addition, I conducted interviews with a dozen sleep clinicians and researchers, some affiliated with the MSDC and others not. I also interviewed sleep technicians, nurses and the family members of disordered sleepers.

In *The Slumbering Masses* and related articles (Wolf-Meyer 2008, 2011, 2012), I have written extensively of intimacy as a way to conceptualise the relationships between individuals and their therapeutic treatments and the doubts that exist between physicians and the science of sleep. Herein, I want to think about these two concerns as discursive and related to the ethnographic representation of cases, operating first between interviewer and interviewee, and secondarily between author and reader. In the case of intimacy, I am interested in how relationships between individuals and material objects and processes alter the capacities of each; as we open ourselves up to the agentive qualities of pharmaceuticals, prosthetics, institutional demands and social relations, our bodies are likewise reconfigured. These subtle reconfigurations of our selves allow for further intimate transformations between our bodies and our environments. Physicians often use vagueness and opacity in the scientific and medical literature to manipulate data to provide alternative explanations for empirical realities; doubt allows for the re-diagnosis of a patient's case, possibly with better therapeutic results. I want to play with doubt as a discursive strategy. For most ethnographic writing, the straightforward presentation of evidence is a technique to allay doubt. It is meant to be convincing in its support of argumentation. But what if doubt is produced in ethnographic writing in order to broaden interpretive possibilities for readers? Doubt might be used analogously to Marshall McLuhan's discussion (1994 [1964]) of 'hot' and 'cold' media to unsettle the authority of the text and reauthorise the power of the reader to make interpretive claims. More abstract presentation of cases might move social science beyond 'cold' texts and towards arguments that move beyond the historical and spatial limitations of the original study. I return to these claims by way of conclusion. I turn first to the initial presentation of Ryan's case, and then represent Jack's and Ryan's cases in the sections that follow.

Disclosure and consequence

When I interviewed him, Ryan had been diagnosed with almost all the conditions that a disordered sleeper could be diagnosed with: narcolepsy, REM (rapid eye movement), behavioural disorder, obstructive sleep apnea, shift work sleep disorder, and a vague circadian rhythm disorder. Despite exhibiting symptoms since childhood, he had decided at age 40 that something might be physiologically wrong with him. And it was only at 48 that he finally sought out diagnosis. At the time of our interview, in his mid-fifties, and inching towards retirement, Ryan had some control of his sleep through a mixture of pharmaceuticals, CPAP technology *(continuous positive airway pressure)* and social arrangements of his working time. 'I work a twelve hour shift,' he told me, 'from six at night until six in the morning, or from six in the morning until six at night.' He is employed by a large power company on the East Coast, working to maintain the integrity of the power grid of a large metropolitan area. His workday consists of him sitting in front of a console for hours at a time, with little change in activity or object of focus. This is dull work, but within his unionised labour force, it is a sought-after position since it does not involve handling any electrical equipment and is therefore not life-endangering.

Because of his various sleep disorders – and workplace problems he narrates presently – at work, he takes Provigil, an alertness-promoting drug. He goes on to explain not only his work situation, but how it renders his sleep as disorderly:

> The longest one shift goes is four days, and then I shift to the nights. And I can have one day off in-between, or eight days off in-between . . . And then there's one week when you have to work relief, where you have to work four hours in the morning, then twelve hours that night, and twelve hours the next day, so my biggest problem is 'when do I take my medication'. If I have to skip it, then I'm more of a zombie . . . I took a letter from my neurologist that said that I need to take a midday nap on each shift, and they sent me home for three weeks without pay while they figured out what to do. They brought me back and said, 'If you take a nap, you're fired.' And this is a company with 12,000 employees. And then I took a letter in that said that if I continue to work without napping, I could endanger myself or others, and with that one they sent me home for three months . . . I was on 'crisis suspension', so I got paid for that one . . . My personal feeling is that they don't want anyone to have any kind of personal accommodation or anything because it will open up a can of worms. [My sleepiness was] troublesome when I was a kid, but the older I get, the harder it gets.

'How do you cope with it?' I asked. 'Napping, and working an eight-hour shift. I think napping works. But my employer treats napping as a personal choice, so that means it's a conduct issue. That's what they believe right now.' Ryan is caught in an especially difficult situation: whether or not he expressly discloses his condition to his employer, his behaviour and work-place performance may lead his managers to suspect some problem. The choice he is faced with is an explicit disclosure of his condition, which may result in workplace discrimination of some sort, or an implicit disclosure through his ongoing workplace behaviours, which may also lead to consequences, but without legal recourses available.

Disclosing their conditions to their employers entails consequences for both Ryan and Jack, in each case shaping both the possibilities of their work lives and their lives beyond work. This limits Jack's ability to make his disclosure, as his secrecy allows him to pursue his profession as he desires; admitting his condition to his supervisors would lead to his immediate dismissal or, at best, a curtailing or transformation of his workplace roles, that is, he would be removed from performing operations. The indignity that this would lead to would be tantamount to Jack not working at all, so foreclosing the possibility of admitting to his condition. Ryan does disclose to his employer the nature of his condition and the medical recommendations that could support his ongoing participation in work but, in consequence, he immediately faces disciplinary action, not for his behaviour, but for the affordances he will require as an employee with special dispensations. Ryan is removed from the workplace, albeit temporarily, so that his employers can ascertain the consequences of making allowances for his workplace require-ments. His is eventually given eight-hour shifts, but he still sneaks out to his car during lunch breaks to take a nap, a compromise that at once treats him like other employees – he will be disciplined if caught napping – and different, as he is only given eight- (rather than twelve-) hour shifts.

The differences in Jack's and Ryan's abilities to disclose their conditions to employers are more an effect of narcissistic attachment than an effect of perceived consequences, although they are clearly entangled with one another. For Ryan, his job is just that: a job. He has risen through the ranks to a position of seniority, is protected by his union, and is waiting for his eventual retirement. Reaching retirement with full benefits is the one fear that his disclosure skirts, but he has his union to protect him from being summarily dismissed. For Jack, the story is different. His attachment to his career extends beyond his position, and it is tied to his understanding of himself as a specialist, extremely capable at what he does: the loss of his job would not simply affect him, but would affect his potential, future patients, who may fall into the care of a less capable heart surgeon. Jack's notion of his standing among his peers may be fanciful, but it is enough justification for him to seek out his colleagues for private consultations, especially when compounded with the most likely outcome of what may happen to him if he were to disclose his condition to his supervisors. Secondarily, his decisions about his career will impact on his family and the lives of those he cares for in a non-professional manner. Part of the difficulty of these disclosures, however, is that despite there being treatments for narcolepsy and other sleep disorders, there is also the acceptance on the part of physicians that none of these treatments is so effective as to render disorderly sleepers into perfectly and predictably orderly ones (Wolf-Meyer 2009).

Elsewhere, I have suggested that contemporary American medicine is characterised by its reliance upon therapy, that is, it depends upon regular, incomplete interventions on individuals in order for the individual to retain a sense of normality and orderliness (Wolf-Meyer 2014). This model of intervention stands in contrast to ideas of cures, which offer one-time, complete resolution of symptoms. While a cure offers the promise of returning an individual to a pre-symptomatic state or a new normality, therapies require constant negotiation between patients and physicians, individuals and treatments (pharmaceuticals, prosthetics, etc.), and between an individual and his or her social obligations. Therapies can change over time, lose effectiveness or become compromised by parallel prescriptions: in so doing, they always risk becoming ineffective. And because therapies are incomplete in their resolution of symptoms, there is also always the possibility that an individual will miss taking a pill or other temporary treatment, resulting in the full return of symptoms. This is part of the underlying problem for both Jack and Ryan. While treatments exist for their disorderly sleep, they are not cures and cannot return Jack and Ryan to normality in a resolute fashion. Instead, for Jack and Ryan, only temporary relief exists, and they will have to risk the possibility of missing a day's medication or the failure of a treatment to prove effective in a time of need. Their conditions are risky for what they might entail in the future, threatening their own and others' lives and wellbeing.

Disclosure once removed

Jack was a test pilot; his professional life has been stressful and competitive. Graduating from university, Jack enlisted in the US Air Force, flying missions in the first Iraq War in the early 1990s. At the time, Jack would experience brief dizzy spells at takeoff, which he came to attribute to lightheadedness associated with the dramatic speeds and changes in altitude he was experiencing. He never talked about it with anyone. When he wasn't flying, Jack would find himself dozing through the day, attributing his perceived laziness to the stresses associated with flying manned missions over a warzone. To offset his drowsiness, he would routinely drink a pot's worth of coffee before and after lunch, cup by cup. But rather than feel wired by the caffeine, Jack still struggled to stay awake. Only during operations did he really feel most engaged with the world around him. Jack came to think of himself as an adrenaline junkie, really only alive when he was under stress and defying death in one form or another. Returning from Iraq, Jack enrolled in martial arts classes, began rock climbing, and found a job for a large military research and design company that specialises in experimental aircraft design. After more than a decade of flying new stealth bombers and fighter jets, his employer offered Jack the opportunity to test its next-generation space shuttle, a low orbit passenger plane intended to ferry high-paying passengers to the edge of space. Leading up to this opportunity, Jack began to realise that what he had convinced himself of – his status as an adrenaline junkie – was a polite fiction which protected him from the reality of his condition. One night, at home on a Sunday, he watched an episode of *60 Minutes* with an interview of a noted neurologist who specialised in sleep-related disorders. One of the patients interviewed was a narcoleptic who narrated his symptoms, which aligned perfectly with Jack's own. Consulting with his family doctor, Jack came to understand that the likelihood of his being able to be medicated for narcolepsy and fly was unlikely, if not impossible. But rather than disclose his condition to his employer, Jack decided to pursue a position in the flight simulation facility, training the next generation of pilots to fly drones and jets in emergency situations, never needing to admit his condition to his employer.

Ryan is a police officer in a medium-sized city on the American East Coast. 'I work a twelve hour shift,' he told me, 'from six at night until six in the morning, or from six in the morning until six at night.' He went on to explain: 'The longest one shift goes is four days, and then I shift to the nights. And I can have one day off in-between or eight days off in-between . . . And then there's one week when you have to work relief, where you have to work four hours in the morning, then twelve hours that night, and twelve hours the next day.' Like many Americans who work shift-work schedules – where they change their work shift from week to week in an effort to maintain some kind of egalitarian sharing of the misery relating to night work – Ryan experiences a number of symptoms that his family doctor refers to as shift-work sleep disorder. That is, Ryan experiences insomnia when he has the time to sleep, and sleepiness when he should be awake – even when he's working during the day. Protected by his union, Ryan cannot be fired from his position on the force, but that does not make his work life any easier. In some respects, it makes it more difficult. If the union was not involved, his seniority would not prove so difficult to manoeuvre, and he might be able to be moved to a less desirable desk job. But, as it is, Ryan is poised to retire in a few years. And, although Ryan knows that those few years will be long ones, he consoles himself with taking naps in his patrol car, as long as his partner manages to stay awake.

Discussing Jack's and Ryan's cases raises questions for ethnographic depictions of individuals in risky situations, particularly those where the lives of others are the ones being endangered. The closer my representation of their cases is to the evidence, the more likely I am to provoke the very consequence that they fear. Even in their first presentation, I abide by contemporary ethnographic practice and render each with pseudonyms and remove identifying information about their actual workplaces. Although it has been several years since they were originally interviewed, and in both cases solutions have been reached by Jack and Ryan and their supervisors, there is still the possibility of some sort of backlash against them by those who might identify them: at least this is the assumption of institutional review boards (IRBs) that approve ethnographic research only when it meets standards in obscuring the identity of respondents. But there is a potential problem here: at least in Jack's case, I was privy to information that could affect the lives of patients, and was ethically bound to not disclose the situation I had observed. By presenting Jack's case to me – among the other staff at the sleep clinic – Dr Richards made me as culpable as the rest of his colleagues. Although a solution to the problem was in the offing without my knowledge, the presentation of the case immediately raised ethical concerns for me, although these were summarily suppressed by the strictures of the IRB approval I laboured under. That is, the IRB approval I already had meant that I need not bother with the ethical quandary: the decision of keeping silent (or at least obscuring the identity of the actors) had already been made for me. Should I be exempt from ethical quandary?

My knowledge of Ryan's sleep disorders might have led me to contact his employer, particularly if I felt that the recommendations he had already been given by physicians were insufficient. In Ryan's case, as much as Jack's, lives were at stake. For Jack, it was the patients before him on the surgery table. For Ryan, it was anonymous citizens, who, during times of emergency, might be at risk. But, again, I was removed from the ethical problems associated with these disclosures, protected by the IRB. Similarly, you, my reader, are exempt from these ethical considerations. If you could infer the identities of these two men, you might be put into the position of disclosure on their behalves. And as my representation of these two cases becomes more fictitious, more abstract in relation to the original evidence, the more likely it becomes that you are able to apply the cases to those around you. Maybe Jack the doctor and Ryan the power company worker are far from your social circle – and maybe so are Jack the test pilot and Ryan the police officer – but the further I remove them from their original situations, the more open the interpretive possibilities become. Maybe Jack was not a doctor at all, nor Ryan a power company worker. Maybe those representations were already fictitious, once removed to preserve Jack's and Ryan's identities and lives.

Tertiary disclosures

Jack is a German Shepherd. He is the great-grandchild of German Shepherds who were bred at Stanford University Sleep Disorder Center to test the genetic prevalence of narcolepsy. All of Jack's great-grandparents, grand-parents and parents experienced narcolepsy symptoms; in their relatively comfortable lives at Stanford's laboratory cum dog ranch, this family of dogs was susceptible to spontaneously falling asleep when excited. Play would often turn into a cascade of napping dogs. Dinner time would often become a comedy of errors as technicians prodded dogs awake to eat the meals so eagerly anticipated. Even casual affection for a dog could result in it dozing off at the feet of its caretaker. Jack was no different, prone to falling asleep at times of heightened emotions. What was different about Jack was this: he was born outside of the laboratory, the first generation of dogs born after the research had been decommissioned. How many generations of narcoleptic dogs do you really need to breed to see the hereditary component of narcolepsy, after all? And so Jack lived his life off-campus. But he was precluded from certain kinds of jobs a dog of his breed might do: no sentry work, no actual shepherding. Instead, Jack was adopted into a nice, suburban family living in nearby Woodside, where he spent most of his days lounging on the back porch or family room couch. Jack's genetic legacy haunts him, however innocuous it might seem. On Wednesdays, when the garbage trucks scour the neighbourhood, Jack rises to bark at them, but quickly lapses into sleep amid his excitement. When the school bus approaches the corner on which the children in the family disembark, Jack often falls asleep, overcome by his excitement at seeing the kids. Jack's human family understands his limitations, and while Jack's being overcome with sleepiness might perturb police officers or farmers who employed him, his suburban family is content with a dog they sometimes find humorous in his excitement turned into spontaneous napping.

Ryan is a physician, a heart surgeon, who practises at a large teaching hospital associated with a nearby university in the American Midwest. When he's attending, he works long days, often twelve hours, but regularly upwards of eighteen, as he tends to take his work home with him and is never far from being able to be called in during an emergency situation. In some respects, Ryan is always on call, burdened by his sense of being the most capable heart surgeon on staff. Even at weekends, he's likely to respond to calls from colleagues, and he hasn't taken a vacation in nearly a decade. But Ryan lives with a great deal of anxiety – having a bundle of sleep-related disorders – and he lives in fear that these will be discovered by his colleagues, patients and administrators. At first he thought his excessive daytime sleepiness was simply the result of his long hours of work. He imagined his intermittent insomnia to be related to stresses associated with work and thought his weight gain and laboured breathing during sleep to be an effect of his slowing, ageing metabolism. But as the science and medicine of sleep matured over the 1990s and early 2000s, he saw a number of patients with disorders similar to his own and came to realise that he too was a disorderly sleeper. If he were to reveal his condition to his supervisors, colleagues or patients, he would surely be barred from performing the surgeries he felt so superior to his colleagues at performing, that he felt so defined him as a professional.

Ryan consulted with one of his colleagues – a neurologist also on staff at his hospital – who he imagined would keep his confidence on these matters. What, Ryan asked, could be done to alleviate his symptoms but allow him to work as he had for the past twenty-five years of his professional life? His colleague, Dr Richards, suggested that he deliver a letter to the administrator who oversaw the pulmonary care department at their hospital, which Richards would prepare with recommendations that would ease Ryan's symptoms without disclosing the nature of his sleep disorders. Richards and Ryan collectively hoped that this tactic would provide the administration with 'plausible deniability' related to Ryan's condition, but would also facilitate Ryan in his professional goals and personal desires for sleep. Ryan reported to me:

> I took a letter from my neurologist that said that I need to take a midday nap on each shift, and they sent me home for three weeks without pay while they figured out what to do. They brought me back and said, 'If you take a nap, you're fired.' And then I took a letter in that said that if I continue to work without napping, I could endanger myself or others and with that one they sent me home for three months . . . I was on 'crisis suspension', so I got paid for that one . . . My personal feeling is that they don't want anyone to have any kind of personal accommodation or anything because it will open up a can of worms.

Doctors have always had the ability to take naps during slow periods of a shift, but what Ryan was asking for was a more bureaucratic dispensation that would allow him to nap even during busy times at the hospital. The administration was unwilling to grant this request, and was infuriated by his collusion with Richards. After conducting an investigation, the hospital offered Ryan the opportunity to retire early, move into administration, or be dismissed. Unable to conceive of a life without work, Ryan moved into administration, far removed from patients, and was able to sneak the occasional nap on the couch in his office into his daily schedule of supervision and meetings.

One way to assess the damage that more fictive representations create is to assume that as the gyre of representation widens, so does the doubt produced in the reader by the text. The gap between fact and fiction that this kind of more fictive presentation creates may disrupt the vital intimacy between author and reader by disturbing the reader's sense of verisimilitude. What if I were to tell you that the first presentation of these cases was the most fictionalised and this last presentation the most factual? Ethnographers often toy with their evidence, changing names and locations: a modest fictive art that readers collectively accept as part and parcel of protecting informants. Ethnographers also render many people into composite characters, sometimes mixing experiences and evidence between two or many real people to tell a more cohesive tale: again, a fiction meant to protect the identities of the many involved. But what is the limit of fiction that a reader might be willing to allow in an effort to elicit the truth of the matters at hand?

Throughout the permutations of Jack's and Ryan's stories, some commonalities remain, particularly the nature of their sleep complaints. That is, I maintain my interest in sleep and its relation to American society, particularly as it makes work especially difficult for Jack and Ryan. But might the story be told otherwise to achieve the same ends, might my ethnographic disclosures be bent further to more fully explore the ethical quandaries of Jack, Ryan, those around them and myself?

The risk in these permutations is that they unsettle my authority and your ability to believe in the cases themselves. Although it is rarely discussed, suspension of disbelief is not something usually attributed to the reader of social scientific writing. We assume implicitly that the events, people and places we read about are real, although we might grant leeway in their representations for ethical considerations. Ethnographic acts of disclosure, particularly of the kind that I present in the introduction to account for the empirical basis for my research and argument herein, are widely accepted as necessary conventions of social scientific writing. As readers, we want to believe the facticity of what is presented to us, although we may question its representativeness or the rigour under which the research was conducted. Breaking from these conventions – not presenting these kinds of background conditions or disclosing too much about one's state of mind or concerns (Behar 2003 [1994], Briggs 1971, Favret-Saada 1981) – is likely to provoke questions about the veracity of the research. That is, too much disclosure on the part of the ethnographer may call into question the ethnographer's ability to faithfully represent what he or she has witnessed, however situated that knowledge is acknowledged to be. But, breaking from these conventions may equally help to ethnomethodologically unsettle the frames of ethnographic writing to the point that the intimacy we desire in our reading practices makes room for the interpretive latitude of doubt we may need to use ethnographic representations of cases in our own lives. The more doubt a text produces, the more applicable it becomes for readers who approach it from different contexts than that of the author; in order to make my discussions of sleep disorders and their complications meaningful to those outside of the world of sleep, some abstraction, some fictionalisation is required. And even for those who are intimately involved in sleep, too literal of a presentation of data means very little – some interpretive room is required to see ourselves in other worlds. A little more doubt may lead to greater textual intimacy, at once asking the reader to interpret the text at hand, but also providing the reader with tools to use in her or his engagement with the world beyond the text.

Disclosure as method

I know a man who drinks the equivalent of three pots of coffee each day. He stretches it out over the course of the day, but he drinks it nonetheless. If you believe that claim, it probably has to do with my demonstrating my sleep expertise throughout this chapter. But if I were to tell you that it was six pots, would that be believable? Would twelve? As Manderson points out in her introduction to this volume, the storytellers, the disclosers, are often put into a position of vulnerability; they are open to claims on the part of their interlocutors about the truthfulness or accuracy of their disclosures, as well as being subject to their interlocutors' reactions to what has been disclosed. Some of the artifice of ethnographic writing – like discussions of sample size, method and the use of generic conventions around the presentation of evidence and the kinds of evidence deployed – are meant to mitigate these vulnerabilities. Despite often trafficking in extreme and exceptional cases, ethnography tends to be accepted as a credulous act, a method that defrays potential disbelief in the cases it presents. Across worlds and experiences that might be very alien to its readers, ethnography gains its power by revelling in the mundane as much as exposing the exceptional. This pairing of the mundane and the extraordinary depends on the use of the realist conventions that Auerbach outlines in the presentations of data: the extraordinary might seem impossible if not for an ordinary foundation. Although ethnographers are exposed to the vulnerabilities of storytelling, they have means – discursive and methodological – to allay disbelief. No reader need begin an ethnography by suspending disbelief, although he or she may come to that position if overly exceptional cases are consistently presented, unmoored from some mundane everyday reality. However, although boring, the mundane is believable: the more exceptional cases become, the more incredible, the less able they are to sustain the belief of the reader, although, in their moment, they may make for compelling reading.

The representations of cases can be moulded away from their empirical basis, but this practice has its limits and, at least in the cases I present here, that limit is history. These limits are the limits of realism though, and are self-imposed: I could wander further in my representations if I were willing to wander deeper into the rhetorical. For me, the aim in my presentation of these cases of disorderly sleep – both here and in my work more generally – is to think through the contortions institutions produce in the human body: what people have to do to align themselves with the expectations of normal everyday life in the USA through the manipulation of their bodies to meet the demands of the institutions with which they interact. So, although I might trade sleep disorders for some other condition, ultimately I must be able to still reach the same conclusions. If that substitution would render the cases more compelling, it might be worth the potential disbelief readers would bring to the text. But, it might mean this text would be something other than ethnographic, and more appropriately thought of as fiction, pure and simple.

The line between fiction and ethnography, however, is a fine one, and when it is muddied, it upsets not simply the text at hand, but generic conventions of documentary representations across disciplines, not solely related to writing.

Nearly thirty years after the critiques of representation that rocked the ethnographic social sciences and anthropology especially, the arts of ethnographic writing no longer seem so explicitly controversial. That this is so may have less to do with the generic conventions of ethnographic writing than it does with the changing expectations of social science readers. Or it may be a balance of the two, relying on changes in writing and reading practices. Writers and readers have become accustomed to particular kinds and degrees of disclosure on the part of ethnographic writers and their interlocutors: too much unsettles a text by making it appear too subjective, too little renders a text inert by inferring a level of objectivity that is not credible. This state of affairs might not be the best for ethnographic writing as it may index growing apathy with regard to ethnographic writing, for writers and readers both. It may index the strictures of the market on social science writing, where more experimental forms of presentation are seen as a market risk rather than a valuable experiment. Whatever the reasons for the decrease of experimental ethnographic writing, ethnographers have at their disposal means to expand the limits of ethnographic writing by experimenting with how and what they disclose, that is, their methods, their knowledge, their interlocutors and the worlds they hope to construct through their ethnographic texts.

Ethnography is fundamentally an ethical practice. This ethical relationship is generally assumed to be between the ethnographer and his or her interlocutors, as the ethnographer works to both be faithful to the experiences of his or her subjects and also works to protect their identities and material, everyday situations. But, given that ethnographic writing now balances the demands of disclosure on the part of writers as well as interlocutors, the ethical relationship embedded in every ethnographic text is fundamentally between writer and reader. One last disclosure, by way of example: during the same period in which I interviewed Ryan and other disordered sleepers, I interviewed a man named Ken. I met Ken through Talk About Sleep (*www.talkaboutsleep.com*), an internet site dedicated to sleep-related support for individuals and their families. Ken was a relatively active member of the community, posting regularly and often responding to other people's posts with his own experiences navigating his anxiety-related insomnia and obstructive sleep apnea. I eventually asked if he would be agreeable to a telephone interview, and we set up a time. Although my life history interviews with disordered sleepers often stretched past an hour and a half, as we discussed their family, school, work, recreational and medical histories, my interview with Ken was a terse eleven minutes. He would answer my questions with one- or two-word answers and never elaborated his answers when prompted. At the end of the interview – which I struggled to stretch out – I felt embarrassed. It was my first real interview failure. But it was not my last. Of the interviews I conducted with disordered sleepers, about 10% of them were equally awkward.

Why have I waited so long to make this disclosure, one that is fundamental to my experience as a researcher and has bearing on the presentation of my data? That social scientists do not regularly admit their failures troubles the veracity of social science claims. If our science is built only upon positive evidence, that is, only built upon success, means that a world of seemingly unasked questions remains, despite answers maybe already existing. That we can choose to admit our failures or not highlights the ethical burden inherent in ethnographic writing; we are always choosing whether to tell the whole truth or only part of it, whatever generic conventions we choose to deploy. Full disclosure may never be possible as a practice of ethnographic writing, but until we come to terms with the powers and limits of disclosure in our writing, we will have yet to reckon with the reflective critiques of the 1980s that challenged – and seemingly continue to challenge – dominant forms of ethnographic representation. Which is all to say: have I disclosed enough?

Note

1   I am indebted here to Christopher Priest's novel *The Affirmation* (Priest 1996 [1981]), in which the protagonist sets about writing his autobiography and finds the factual presentation of his life to lack truth; only by rendering it increasingly fantastic is he able to get to the truth of his experiences. By the end of the novel, it is unclear whether his initial presentation of reality is factual or if that was the fiction he created.

8 Transsexual women's strategies of disclosure and social geographies of knowledge

Muriel Vernon

For transsexual women, disclosure, or revealing one's transsexual status to others, has been a central moral concern since transsexualism became recognised as a legitimate psycho-medical condition in the 1950s (Benjamin 1966, Green and Money 1969). Transsexual individuals' disclosure models and strategies can vary greatly; however, all acts of disclosure carry a moral undertone which mediates why, when, how and to whom transsexual women reveal all, none or some aspects of their differently gendered past. 'The decision to be "out" as trans', notes Catherine Connell, 'is one that must be individually negotiated based on a number of complex and sometimes contradictory financial, psychological, political, and personal considerations' (2010: 38). Constructing moral personhood thus figures prominently in how transsexual women present themselves to and interact with their social worlds.

In this chapter, exploring the decisions and processes of disclosure among transsexual women, I use a particular lexicon. Although transsexual identities are generally subsumed in the larger category of transgender (or simply 'trans') identities, most transsexuals unambiguously identify as either men or women and usually express and pursue a desire for permanent hormonal and surgical body modification. Transgender individuals, on the other hand, may present greater gender ambiguity, and may not or only partially express and pursue such desires. Transgender as a categorical description of gender non-conformity can also include variations of genderqueer, genderfluid or non-binary gender identities. Even so, many scholars use the terms transgender and transsexual interchangeably, or simply refer to transsexuals as transgender to indicate a more inclusive or progressive understanding of identity construction. I prefer, however, to differentiate these terms, both because my ethnographic data for this chapter focuses on individuals who have undergone hormonal and genital reassignment, and because the category of transgender can subsume any and all gender variance for a multitude of personal and political reasons. I also use the word *cissexual* (the latin prefix 'cis' indicating the concept of matching or being on the same side), in contrast to transsexual, to refer to non-transsexual persons in a more neutral manner than presenting non-transsexuality as 'normal', 'non-pathological' or 'unmarked'.

Drawing on ethnographic fieldwork with transsexual women undergoing genital reassignment surgery (GRS) in 2010,[1] in this chapter I contextualise how transsexual women's moral concerns of their dishonesty and deception, as perceived by cissexuals, are negotiated against the simplistic binary of being 'out' (disclosure) or 'stealth' (non-disclosure). Drawing on anthropological theories of morality, especially the work of Jarrett Zigon, which I discuss further below, I argue against the assumption that non-disclosure is dishonest or deceptive, by challenging the moral reasoning that equates disclosure with a socially shared idea of truth. In transsexual disclosures, two opposing moral models are at work, each representing different notions of what constitutes one's 'true gender'. These opposing moral models, when evoked in disclosure contexts between cissexual and transsexual individuals, lead to what Jarrett Zigon calls 'a moral breakdown' (2007), bringing about what I would call a relational rupture. In these relational ruptures, transsexual women's claim that their gender is as 'true' and 'real' as that of natal women is often negated by cissexuals, who maintain a discursive and conceptual boundary between cissexual and transsexual genders, by anchoring transsexual genders in natal sex and gendered socialisation.

I substantiate my argument by complicating disclosure as a moral directive towards a shared understanding of transsexual identities. I suggest that disclosure is not an achievement by a person towards a shared ethos of honesty but, rather, it is a social expectation of aligning with hegemonic or dominant discursive understandings of gendered truth. This perspective illuminates how morality constructs its objects of truth, by demanding that acts of disclosure align with or conform to a shared cultural understanding of truth. Disclosure as an obligatory practice of truth alignment with gender as an ascribed, not achieved identity is most problematic here, and not the disclosure binary of being out or not.

Transsexual disclosure past and present

In the 1950s, the goal of gender transition was to enable transsexuals to present as ordinary men and women, and utilise stereotypical, coherent, gender-normative life histories which were believable and escaped scrutiny by others (Meyerowitz 2002). The first transsexuals treated by psychiatric and medical specialists accordingly were advised and presumed to desire to live in 'stealth'[2] once their social and medical transition had concluded. The moral implications of this model were rarely questioned.[3] These concerns are now central as transsexualism has developed from an understudied psychopathology to a globally recognised, self-acclaimed identity and growing community. Many transsexual women themselves have taken moral issue with the prescriptive stealth model for various reasons.[4] But the most salient reason is essentially articulated in moral dispositionality: non-disclosure of a transsexual status is legally and morally interpreted as deception and dishonesty, and many transsexual women struggle with the notion of disclosure while desiring to present their 'true selves'[5] to the world.

Since the shared cultural ethos of voluntary self-disclosure rests on honesty about the self, transsexual women devise culturally distinct strategies and narratives of disclosure to accommodate this expectation. In these practices, transsexual women must balance disclosure of information about their differently gendered past while convincingly presenting their current gender identities as 'real' and 'true'. Because of the anticipatory notion of societal rejection or invalidation of their current gender identities, transsexual women's disclosure practices are invariably informed by abiding with a 'common sense' morality based on honesty. But they are also informed by authentic presentations of 'true selves' as honest selves, whereby moral personhood is enacted and balanced with authenticity of selfhood. While most cissexuals would argue that the 'true' gender of transsexuals is based on their natal sex and past gender socialisation, many transsexuals argue that they have always felt themselves to be or belong to the opposite gender, and that this confirms their 'true' gender. Transsexual women thus face an ongoing moral dilemma of how to disclose their differently gendered past while sustaining credibility of their current gender in their social lives.

Common-sense morality and contexts of disclosure

Assuming that transsexuals and cissexuals share a 'common sense' morality that idealises enduring honesty codes, morality is nonetheless an ongoing process of both reproducing and challenging social relations (Robbins 2009, 2007, Turner 2003b, Zigon 2009, 2007). 'Rather than being found in the moral beacon of a transhistorical, transcultural "common moral sense"', writes Turner (2003b: 209), 'the common morality that exists in American laws, public policies, and social institutions requires proponents to engage in the work of debating, persuading, and outmaneuvering those individuals with alternative moral claims.' However, even if honesty codes can be agreed upon as part of a shared value system, this does not mean a shared moral interpretation of what constitutes honesty. Turner adds that '[s]uch a historical, "local" version of common morality is also a morality of power, insofar as laws, policies, and social institutions promote the interests of some parties, while blocking the goals and substantive concerns of others. This revised concept of the common morality means that not everyone, everywhere holds it in common' (2003b: 209).

Jarrett Zigon reiterates this claim by adding that morality is 'essentially a social mode of being' (2007: 135), while also favouring a 'local' vantage point to understand morality. Zigon's definition of morality reiterates Turner's definition, in that '[m]orality can be considered as three different, but certainly interrelated, aspects that are themselves pluralistic: (1) the institutional; (2) that of public discourse; and (3) embodied dispositions'

(2009: 258). The latter part is of particular interest in transsexual disclosure contexts, because '[m]orality as embodied dispositions is one's everyday way of being in the world' (260). Taking issue with moral dispositions as unreflective, Zigon argues that these become rather open modes of being in 'certain difficult relationship situations within which one might find oneself' (2007: 137). Such situations cause what he calls a 'moral breakdown' which brings about a 'moment in which ethics must be performed.' This leads him to make a distinction between 'morality as the unreflective mode of being-in-the-world and ethics as a tactic performed in the moment of the break-down of the ethical dilemma' (137). 'In other words,' he continues, 'when an individual finds him- or herself in a moment of moral breakdown, that person also finds that a demand is being placed upon him or her ... The ethical demand, then is a product of a particular situation and the individuals involved. Therefore, the ethical demand is a situationally sensitive and, thus, a social demand' (138).

I take Zigon's moral breakdown necessitating an ethical moment as the constitutive antecedent of what, in this chapter, I call a relational rupture. I use this term to refer to the discursive effect of diverging moral disposi-tions which may disrupt personal relationships. I argue that in moments of relational rupture, moral dispositionality becomes most salient, requiring conscious repair to restore a shared sense of morality within relationships. For a transsexual woman, disclosure contexts put in motion a conscious dilemma of presenting herself to the world if it can be anticipated that she will be discredited from here on. When a relational rupture results from voluntary or involuntary disclosure, an interpersonal ethical violation of presenting oneself 'untruthfully' occurs, necessitating relational repair. Individuals thus experience what Zigon calls an 'ethical moment' which 'occurs when some event or person intrudes into the everyday life of a person and forces her to consciously reflect upon the appropriate ethical response' (2009: 262). In this context, transsexual women must offset the default disclosure notion of 'untruthfulness', by articulating their current gender identities as 'true' and morally sound. But while Zigon argues that these moments of ethics are creative moments, 'for by performing ethics, persons create, even if ever so slightly, new moral personhoods and enact new moral worlds' (262), this goal is often difficult to achieve intersubjectively in transsexual disclosure contexts.

Even if transsexual disclosure appears to be the 'right thing to do', performing ethical personhood (i.e. the revelation of a transsexual identity) is nonetheless complicated. Even though transsexualism may be factual, it conflicts with performing authentic personhood. And although morality is enacted by adhering to a common sense understanding of honesty, for a transsexual woman the shared meaning of honesty conflicts with her gendered self-perception as being honest to herself. For the cissexual person, the common-sense understanding of honesty also jeopardises his or her moral personhood because disclosed honesty obligates a reward of acceptance as part of moral performance, while at the same time he or she may feel averse to now knowing about the person's transsexual status or past. This situation also exemplifies Zigon's ethical moments because they 'occur when for one reason or another the range of possible moralities available do not adequately "fit" the context. In these breakdowns a shift of consciousness occurs in which a person or persons must consciously and creatively find a way to be moral' (263). The situational 'demand' of the other, in achieving or reconstituting a moral basis of a social relationship, again requires conscious action before a return to any 'unreflective' everydayness of moral life is possible.

Disclosure situations exemplify not only situations of conflict where moral personhood takes primacy, but also situations steeped in recent cultural change, including in the context of the emergence of transsexual personhood. Before the possibility of transsexual personhood entered human cognitive schemas about gender, Garfinkel's 'natural attitude'[6] that there are only two sexes and two genders, and that both sex and gender are ascribed not achieved, and are therefore immutable from birth onwards, predominated our understanding of one of the most basic aspects of human life. Transsexual personhood, however, puts these concepts into question, in both theory and practice. But while some transgender-identified individuals purposefully intend to upset or reject this gender binary and the hierarchy it creates (Davis 2008), many transsexuals attempt to assimilate into the binary by reproducing the social norms pertaining to genders rather than challenging them. They do so, however, from what I call a 'transcentric' moral positionality which underscores the subjectivity of claiming a gender. This functions in opposition to a 'ciscentric' moral positionality that denies gender as something which can be changed, achieved, or subjectively claimed.

Transcentric vs. ciscentric moral models

Transcentric vs. ciscentric moral models exemplify distinctly moral positions because simple 'essentialist' vs. 'constructivist' positions are neither culturally and historically neutral, nor apolitical. Ciscentric models here represent dominant moralities expressed in the 'right to know' which frames non-disclosure of one's transsexual status as harmful and dishonest. Non-disclosure, for example, is often used as a legal reason for marriage annulment and in so-called 'trans-panic'[7] defence cases. Beauchamp notes:

> Cultural representations of gender variant people depend on the popular notion that with enough scrutiny, one's 'true' gender can be revealed at the level of the body . . . The constant repetition of this narrative structure locates violence not in the institutional practices of media, medicine or law, or in the gender-normative behaviors and relationships they enforce, but instead in individual trans people's apparently fraudulent personal lives. Echoing this perspective, legal cases dealing

with violence against gender variant individuals often revolve around the victim's responsibility to disclose their trans status or birth-assigned sex. Such cases imply or outright claim that the individual's dishonest concealment of their 'true' sex was the root cause of the violent actions taken against them.

(Beauchamp 2009: 358)

At first, the legal and medical processes which legitimise a transsexual person's change of gender seem to contradict ciscentric morals by supporting laws which recognise transsexuals' subjective sense of gender. But this magnifies rather than diminishes the ciscentric notion of anchoring a person's 'true' gender in the past. The higher the effort of legal and medical conceal-ment, the greater the perceived harm in non-disclosure and the higher the moral offence to perceived deception. Because medical records and clinical language in particular implement a distinct jargon in describing a trans-sexual's developmental trajectory as 'pre-operative', 'post-operative' or 'non-operative' (and other terms used to describe hormonal effects), transsexuals cannot really extricate themselves from medical subjectivity which must pre-cede (trans)gender subjectivity. As Beauchamp notes, '[m]edical surveillance focuses first on individuals' legibility as transgender, and then, following medical interventions, on their ability to conceal any trans status or gender deviance' (2009: 357).

While legal and medical documents hold a highly validating meaning to transsexual women, once a person's change of gender is known, no legal or medical document confirming the legitimacy of current gender can offset the notion of its apparent artifice. In fact, it would be pointless to show legal documentation with cherished 'F' markers to cissexuals if a transsexual woman's 'real' gender is already in question. Thus, while such legal and medical documents are undoubtedly legitimate and legitimating, some trans-sexual women remain forever stuck in illegitimacy, having effected the legal necessity of these documents in the first place. The contradiction here illum-inates the fact that, again, the more legitimacy transsexuals wish to have as women legally and medically, the greater the institutional need to disclose their transsexualism. And while the law has conscious knowledge of and a contributing role in transsexuals 'passing' as women, it still supports the moral obligation of transsexuals to disclose because of the assumed non-consenting or non-approving attitude of most cissexuals. Beauchamp reiterates this in writing that 'the interplay of medical, legal and cultural representations of transgender populations works to associate the notion of transgender identity with that of secrecy, precisely because it is always understood that the secret can and will eventually be discovered' (358).

Transcentric models, on the other hand, prioritise non-disclosure as a person's 'right to privacy' which is informed by essentialising narratives about deeply existential feelings of always having been the opposite gender. In other words, many cissexuals feel that non-disclosure is deceitful and dishonest, while transsexuals feel that non-disclosure equates with presenting one's 'true' or 'authentic' self to others. The concept of non-disclosure as harmful illuminates ciscentric and transcentric moral cross roads. Sharpe (2012) makes the argument that, from a legal perspective, non-disclosure of gendered histories in marital contexts is already assumed to constitute harm because it assumes that cissexuals would not consent to sexual or marital relations with transsexuals.[8] This makes the law appear inherently transphobic: the cissexual person's 'right to know' takes primacy over the transsexual person's 'right to privacy'. This position proposes that disclosure *must* take place because of the presumed uncertainty of the cissexual person's acceptance and, by extension, it confirms the general notion that transsexual women are 'not really women' in other interactive contexts. Sharpe also questions whether the perceived 'harm' of non-disclosure constitutes any actual or potential experience of the individual, or whether the perceived harm is based in the social conceptions of relationships between cissexuals and transsexuals. Furthermore, ciscentric moral positionality 'suggests that the paramount truth about gender status resides not in the present but in the past. In this sense, failure to reveal the past is presented as inconsistent with the truth and therefore as ethically suspect' (2012: 50). Trans women themselves have commented on the implicitness of taking

> cisgender identity, experience, and perspective as not only supremely and infallibly normative, but also as the yardstick by which ethics and morality themselves are determined. It extends cis privilege into the concepts of 'right' and 'wrong' itself [sic], determining morality primarily by how it relates to a cis person's experience of a conflict, cis perceptions of identity, cis perceptions of 'truth' and 'falsehood', cis perceptions of what are the salient issues in identity and sexual interaction, etc.
>
> (Reed 2012)

The cissexual person's 'right to know' implies that transsexual women are 'not really women' but de facto have (a) the right to legal documentation legitimating a change of gender, and (b) the right to protect their medical history or information. Because of this, transcentric moral models are often supported by the defense that transsexualism is not a primary identifier, but a central and defining aspect of one's personal and private medical history. Transsexual histories as private medical histories build dynamically on bioethics that prioritise confidentiality, beneficence and non-malificence, and aim to protect the individual's autonomy over, and rights to, his or her body (Kleinman 1999, Marshall 1992, Muller 1994, Turner 2003a). For many transsexual women, withholding medical history information is not an act of deception because it conforms to cultural norms which allow for it; nonetheless, the conflation of medical problem and social personhood in the case of transsexualism is more difficult to contend with because of the difficulty of reframing a change of gender as a depersonalised medical problem. This is evident in that the medical capital of individual trans-formation does not easily translate into the cultural capital of social accept-ance, nor does the legal and medical confirmation of gender transition justify rejecting the trans modifier in identity claims and thereby circumventing the moral obligation to disclose. Zigon also reiterates this notion, arguing that 'all institutions, to some extent, consist of a range of moral positions that are debated and contested from within. Despite this internal debate, institutions usually and for the most part publicly articulate a morality *as though* it were internally unquestioned' (2009: 258, emphasis in original).

However, ciscentric and transcentric moral models share a consensus that increasing closeness and intimacy also increase the need for disclosure, even if all disclosures within relationships are ideals and not always realities. Almost all of my participants, when asked about when, whether and how disclosure happens in intimate contexts, reiterated this notion one way or another. For example, one participant said 'I would have to disclose to a potential spouse as I wouldn't want to be emotionally invested in a close relationship only to have them find out and then start hating me for being a transgender.' Another bluntly noted, 'If you wait too long, you're likely to fuck up the relationship.' The rising moral obligation to disclose also reiterates, as Talia Bettcher notes, that 'intimate personhood is profoundly moral in nature' (2012: 324). Her claim that 'genitalia are fundamental to the moral structure of the intimate body' because they 'morally complete' the body (326) speaks strongly not only to the desires of transsexual women to complete the body-self by means of genital reassignment surgery, but also to present a body-self that is recognisable to heteronormative frameworks of gendering and sexualisation. The very fact that this is a conscious endeavour, and not a natural or 'given' completion, artificialises the process in lieu of the given social history of the transsexual body, with the intent of erasing or hiding it from both intimate sexual and moral scrutiny. How then do transsexual women negotiate this dilemma of disclosing their differently gendered past while retaining the credibility of their current gender? Drawing on my own research participants' disclosure strategies, I identified two distinct practices: the first I call creating *social geographies of knowledge*; the second is what a participant called a *language of exclusion*.

Social geographies of knowledge

Social geographies of knowledge can mean creating a geographical separa-tion of social circles and it can mean creating a cognitive separation of social circles based on interpersonal closeness, which help transsexual women compartmentalise who knows what about them. The compartmentalisation of knowledge dissemination is of course not unique to transsexual women. However, from their initial 'coming out' phases to post-transition life, transsexual women contend with cost-benefit analyses of disclosure that are much more complex than the adoption of a dichotomous 'out' or 'closeted' identity. For example, one of my research participants devised a strategy of disclosure based on local knowledge. She said 'If you're from Michigan, you know I'm trans; if you're trans then you know I'm trans; if you're from California and you're not trans, then you don't know that I'm trans … except for one person.' But like many others, she harboured a constant worry about involuntary disclosure at work. 'That's the one problem with being stealth,' she said, '… effectively, you're hiding, you're hiding a part of yourself, and so if it gets out at work that I am trans, then that's going to completely change my, that work dynamic, that social, professional social dynamic will be completely changed.' She often thought of the consequences of involuntary outing: 'I do envision different treatment so, like people being less willing to help in certain situations, less inclusion in female spaces. I would expect an extreme othering from the male population.' On the other hand, remaining a resident in their hometown also anchors transsexual women's transition experience into the context of their past local lives. As another participant illustrated, 'I live in the city I grew up in, so my past life is always around the next corner.' This means that for her, neither living in stealth nor selective non-disclosure was a viable option.

Similar distinctions of compartmentalised knowledge were drawn between work and social networking sites. While employment environments often constituted stealth spaces, as many transsexual women feared detrimental consequences of being out at work, social networking webpages were often revelatory spaces of disclosure. For instance, in contrast to being stealth at work, a participant posted to everybody on Facebook that she was undergoing genital reassignment surgery. While walking dangerously close to involuntary disclosure, she avoided thinking about what would happen if a co-worker tried to 'friend' her. Work spaces generally constitute more difficult disclosure environments for transsexuals because of highly policed gendered bathroom arrangements and changing room segregation, and the often covert assigning of gender-typical, everyday office tasks to women or men respectively (e.g. women make coffee, men do more heavy lifting). A significant number of my participants who were 'out' had experienced barriers to gender appropriate bathroom use, changing room use, and social inclusion in gendered activities at the work place. Those who did not experience any problems either worked at companies with highly inclusive LGBT (lesbian, gay, bisexual, transgender) employment protection, or simply did not disclose their transsexual status (at least not to their immediate co-workers; HR personnel generally know of the past history of transsexual staff by way of legal document paper trails).

Casual sexual or long-term relationships were equally difficult to negotiate into social geographies of knowledge (disclosure) because delayed or involuntary telling could lead to violence and rejection; here the anticipatory notion of a relational rupture was quite salient. On one hand, as one participant put it, involuntary disclosure can 'get you hurt', but voluntary disclosure can 'send people running before they even get to know you', or, as another participant claimed, 'put weird ideas about "what's down there" into [people's] minds'. But while the consensus on intimacy and sexual relationship followed the logic of Bettcher and others who argue that increasing closeness necessitates disclosure, here again lines were invariably drawn around ciscentric 'right to know' moral models which in turn produce the common fears of violence and rejection. One common strategy of 'feeling out' whether a potential partner has adverse views on transsexuals was an 'if/then' approach, based on the belief that people who generally have positive attitudes towards the LGBT community would be more accepting of a person's transsexualism or differently gendered past. In this case, an over-preparedness for a relational rupture based on disclosure conditioned how and when transsexual women revealed this information to others.

As noted, 'trans-panic' defence cases, in which cissexuals 'discovered' the 'true sex' of their pre-operative transsexual partners and reacted violently upon such discovery, are neither rare nor novel; such cases can be said to inform much of the popular folklore of transsexuals 'duping' cissexuals into sexual encounters. But this ignores the difficulty of finding the right time and words to bring up one's transsexual status (pre- or post-operatively) to sexual partners, because it is not always possible or convenient. This is especially evident when negotiating sexual safety. For instance, Kosenko notes that trans people often 'fear losing out on the validation that comes from sex in the transgender role' (2010: 8) and that generally, 'the lack of language with which to talk about transgender bodies and sex acts limited their ability to create shared meaning and to achieve their sexual safety goals in relationships' (9). Most participants also justified not disclosing when the encounter was anticipated to be purely sexual and singular. The perceived immorality of purely sexual encounters in and of themselves appeared to justify non-disclosure. But almost all narratives about the compartmentalisation of information carried a connotation of lying, hiding and secrecy, which made for consistent dilemmas in disclosure contexts.

Creating social geographies of knowledge thus correlates to actual local and cognitive mapping. This makes compartmentalising knowledge, and withholding knowledge from others about one's transsexual status, a distinctly moral project. The notion of compartmentalising information about oneself is already implicitly moral in that it prioritises withholding rather than disclosing. That which is withheld is assumed to be of some expected adverse consequence to the discloser, which is reiterated in the data above. From the perspective of the receiver of such information, however, disclosure also produces compartmentalisation dilemmas in that knowledge of transsexualism transforms perceptions of a person's 'true' gender permanently. This is because to recognise someone's unambiguous status as 'woman' requires not only cognitive work, but also enacting a moral ethos of acceptance based on honesty. Moreover, when the receiver of disclosed information about a differently gendered past acknowledges the transsexual person's current gender and the desire to live in stealth, he or she, too, must navigate these social geographies alongside the transsexual person – he or she thus becomes 'stealth by proxy'. This sometimes creates a moral burden for cissexuals and transsexuals alike. For example, my own research participants included individuals who were grandparents. Contexts in which the grandchild had no knowledge of the grandparent's transsexual status and interacted with them as 'grandmothers' rather than 'grandfathers' were problematic for cissexual family members who still saw their child's 'grandmother' as their own father. Explaining to children that 'grandma' was also 'daddy's dad' became a complicated manoeuvre of redefining kinship roles, and a unique moral dilemma for families with transsexual members. These examples show that the stealth/out binary is hardly a firm boundary, but rather subject to constant situational negotiation. As one participant noted, 'as a transsexual you come out probably for the rest of your life'.[9]

A language of exclusion

Operating from a transcentric moral position, many transsexual women present themselves to the world as their 'true' or 'authentic' selves. True selves here convey the private and subjective experience and conviction of having always been or having belonged to the opposite gender (Mason-Schrock 1996). However, many realised the following dilemma to 'disclose "who one is" and come out as a pretender or masquerader, or refuse to disclose (be a deceiver) and run the risk of forced disclosure, the effect of which is exposure as a liar' (Bettcher 2007: 50). To circumvent the notion of non-disclosure as deception, many transsexual women use what one participant termed 'a language of exclusion' to capitalise on the common notion that people 'fill in the blank' when segments of personal histories are not disclosed explicitly. For example, when talking about childhoods, almost all participants chose gender-neutral phrases such as 'when I was little', 'when I was young' or 'when I was a child'. Only one participant (out of fifty in total) chose to say 'when I was a little boy' and only seven other participants chose to say 'when I was a little girl'. One common modifier of when or whether participants adjusted or neutralised gendered pronouns, however, depended on the social context or situation. If childhoods were talked about in the presence of individuals who had knowledge of participants' past lives, participants were more likely to use neutral or masculine pronouns to refer to themselves. If, however, the company was mixed (i.e. only some people knew), the neutral or feminine gender pronouns predominated.

In terms of referring to their current or former spouses, about half of my participants would either say 'ex' or 'spouse' or 'partner' instead of 'wife' or 'ex-wife'. Only two participants would explicitly say 'ex-wife'. On the other hand, only two participants chose to deliberately 're-gender' their former wives or girlfriends, or 're-gender' the relationship. For example, one participant's ex-wife was now 'just an old girlfriend' and she did not dwell on the details of their relationship or recreate a new narrative. If anything, she said she would omit details so as to not lie about the legally distinctive aspect of heterosexual marriage. Another participant re-gendered 'ex-wives' to 'ex' and 'ex-spouse' and used male pronouns. She had also changed all of her ex-wives' names to male names. Conversely, most participants who were parents chose to say 'parent' over 'father' and some would occasionally say 'my child's birthmother' or 'my child's other mother', indexing a lesbian relationship. No participant chose to say 'mother' instead of 'father', which curiously reveals a unanimous hesitation (or perhaps a cultural 'taboo' specific to trans women) to modify traditional kinship roles and terminology to accommodate a change of gender within the family structure. This finding was also confirmed by a complementary lack of insistence by participants to be called 'mom' by their children, regardless of age.

Other distinctly gendering traits, activities or events, often omitted from or modified in narratives of past lives, included a variety of topics, leaving either blanks in stories or filling these with gendered substitutes. For example, one participant joked, 'I don't care what they cut off, I still like football', but she would omit mention of having actually played football when she was young. Another participant would say she had a military career but adjust the story to reflect a co-ed environment, and yet another omitted military details like being drafted. Others would omit phases of sexual experimentation, male–male rape, and drag performance. One participant modified 'oil field stories' as she felt these were clear 'give aways' to the all-male nature of her work, placing these into a third-person narrative. Other common omissions included being an altar boy, choirboy or busboy because female analogues to these are linguistically and culturally non-existent. A few participants tried to omit and avoid talk about all gendering contexts in the past, and almost all participants favoured gendered neutrality in recounting professional or personal experiences of their lives.

Although most participants did not feel that 'un-gendering' themselves to efface gender neutrality constituted deception or dishonesty per se, consciously 're-gendering' themselves as well as former or current partners or previous relationships was perceived by some as deceptive. Most notably, however, the degrees of stealth and outness did *not* determine whether participants chose gender-neutral terms to talk about themselves in disclosure contexts. This preference for gender neutrality in personal history narratives reveals a heightened concern for moral personhood achieved through balancing gender legitimacy and a coherent life history.

While classic models of stealth presume that transsexual women retro-actively create female analogues to their male life histories, modern models of *both* being stealth and being out are based on creating gender neutral pasts. The difference between re-gendering and un-gendering one's past complicates binaries of disclosure vs. non-disclosure because un-gendering one's past mediates moral concerns of transsexual women's integrity of self-presentation. There are not only different forms of morality, but also different forms of truth-telling at work. As Zigon remarks, '(t)ruth-telling and lying are situationally negotiated, questioned, and worked-through in different ways by different persons within and beyond this social context. There is no dominant value that persons feel compelled to follow, but rather there is a range of possibilities for morally and ethically acting' (2009: 273).

Moral confirmation and denial of authentic selfhood

Ciscentric and transcentric moral models reveal a critical limitation of moral aspects to disclosure because disclosure presumes 'passing' as in not being read as transsexual. Passing is an already paradoxical notion because it denotes that only those who already know of a person's transsexual status could determine whether transsexuals could pass or not. If someone passes, they are engaged in performative acts which are intended and prove to be so convincing as to obscure their very effort to unknowing audiences. This in turn would erase the recognition of passing. Passing implies some transparency of even the most convincing performance.

However, cissexuals still expect 'visible' or 'outed' or 'non-passing' transsexuals to deliver disclosure narratives about themselves, i.e. confirm or align with what others can perceive or know. The confessional pressure exerted upon transsexuals by cissexuals shows that the perceived transgression is not in *avoiding* discovery by others, but in preventing the *confirmation* of discovery by others. In other words, to insist on a different truth about one's gender *audaciously* challenges the social consensus on who is 'really a woman' because it provokes deeply internalised cultural anxieties about distinguishing real from fake, natural from artificial and, ultimately, truth from deception. While it seems that moral ideals of presenting 'who one really is' are socially rewarded under the honesty ethos of disclosure, transsexuals appear to be excluded from such a privilege as only cissexual genders are real, natural and therefore morally sound. Implementing Zigon's anthropological theory of morality, we can see here that what causes a 'moral breakdown' is not dishonesty per se, but is the insistence on a phenomenological experience of the self independent of a socially agreed upon 'truth'. This relational rupture then is not about a deliberate act of gender *deception*, but rather about a deliberate act of gender *perception* which clearly departs from the social consensus. While transsexual women try to construct themselves as both moral and authentic beings in a cissexual world, this example once more illuminates the ciscentric – and ultimately ethnocentric – assumption that gender immutability is and remains the only truth about gender.

As Zigon (2009) remarks, 'an adequate anthropological theory of moralities must be able to account for both the moral world of a society as well as that of the individuals who live in that society'. Transsexual disclosure contexts exemplify the complexity of such theorisation because, as

Zignon notes, 'a range of possibilities always exists for persons to utilise in their attempt to overcome moral questioning' (2009: 257). However, the confessional pressure to align with ciscentric moral models of what constitutes one's true self shows that it is not necessarily the subjectivity of claiming a gender which is denied, but the impossibility of claiming one is 'just' a woman now. This aspect greatly limits the transsexual women's possibilities to overcome moral questiong. What also remains obscured amidst these moral possibilities is that the legal and medical authority that facilitates constructing womanhood is the same. In situations of conflict, this works ultimately against constructing moral personhood for transsexual women. This is because despite the distinctly symbolic rationales evident in the medico-legal discourse, aiming to make 'undetectable' social inclusion as women possible, the potential for detectability and thus the potential for relational ruptures is not only retained, but defended as a 'right to know' in the law.

Since the contention over what constitutes one's 'true' gender is central to moral breakdowns and relational ruptures in disclosure situations, the point of moral offence takes place at the discursive articulation of identities. For instance, as opposed to unambiguous *transsexual* identities, sometimes *transgender* identities are constructed as a conscious effort to offset the gender binary politically. This means that sometimes the claim to identity is intentionally constructed as 'trans' and not 'just a woman'. In this case, no moral offence to the shared consensus of gender should occur because both sides would acknowledge a violation to the gender 'norm'. But when trans-sexual women lay claims to social and moral equality with natal, cissexual women and refuse to adopt an identifier of differentiation, as they perceive none, a moral breakdown occurs and the potential for relational rupture increases. This is because the conscious rejection of a trans identifier is sometimes interpreted to be just as political as the conscious adoption of a trans identifier. Commenting about identity as a political and by extension moral project, lesbian feminists in particular take issue with the essentialising aspect of transsexual women's identity. For example, Ruby and Mantilla explain that '[i]f identity is held as a given, it is off-limits to criticism or analysis . . . Identity politics is a stealth maneuver that demands, in the name of tolerance, that others do not challenge my politics' (2000: 5). Implicit in this statement, discourse about the self seems to contend with narratives entangled in essentialism and constructivism as moral bases for articulating selfhood.

'True selves' as 'moral selves'

As I have already noted, it is only through legal, medical and popular narratives which reiterate gender as *either* essential and fixed, *or* as fluid and changeable, that moral positions on this matter can form in the first place. Since disclosure is a distinctively moral obligation no matter the perceivable degree of 'stealth' or 'outness', it is also an obligation to narrate oneself into social contexts. Transsexual identities always remain to be explained. These 'explanations' about the self must come about in culturally distinct ways that are firmly bound to narrative as the primary resource of intelligible identity construction. The notion that narratives about the self are dynamically structured cultural practices has been theorised and explicated at length (Bruner 1997, Gergen and Gergen 1983, Sobo 1997). As Sobo notes, 'the narrative construction of oneself as a culturally respectable and moral being is a collaborative intersubjective process' (1997: 9), which presumes that a shared understanding of 'real' or 'true' selves underlies such endeavours. And while 'true selves' correspond to persons acting according to closely held values and a stable sense of authenticity, Mason-Schrock notes that the concept of a true self is a 'nonanalytic label for experience rather than a psychological entity', which nonetheless constitutes 'a powerful fiction' (1996: 177).

Transsexual narratives of the self are particularly interesting in disclosure contexts as they exemplify the necessity not only for an intersubjective collaborative effort, but also for cultural embedding and story patterns (Mason-Schrock 1996). 'Crafting selves,' note Schrock and Reid, 'is an essential form of identity work' (2006: 75). I have previously discussed how information about one's differently gendered past is managed and controlled by implementing social geographies of knowledge and a language of exclusion, and how these are primarily informed by moral concerns. But another important point to consider in analyses of transsexual self-narratives within the moral interface is how the body is incorporated into presentations of authenticity while maintaining moral personhood. If sexual aspects of the body are central to disclosure contexts, for instance whether or not transsexual women have undergone genital reassignment surgery (GRS), then the ubiquitous metaphor of being 'born in the wrong body' prevails in narratives. These narratives existentialise the true self of having always been or already belonging to the other gender, building on contemporary notions of the 'body as a situation' (de Beauvoir 1961) in which the body eventually conforms to the mind through medical intervention and body-self alignment. Here, transsexual subjectivity relies strongly on medical justification and legitimacy of transsexualism as an officially recognised psychopathology and/or medical problem as classified in the *Diagnostic and Statistical Manual of Mental Disorders* (DSM). Medicalisation of gender variance has long been critiqued as pathologising human diversity, yet it helps transsexuals narratively construct moral personhood by distancing the condition away from choice or voluntary deviance. Although a significant number of my own participants retained a 'trans' modifier in their identity construction and presentation, most rejected the trans label, especially after having undergone GRS which unanimously symbolised 'completion' and becoming 'whole selves', the primary purpose of which enabled subjects to represent a more 'authentic' self to the world (Vernon 2012).

It would be rather easy to point out that the problem of discrediting transsexual women's identities in disclosure contexts rests on discursive essentialist notions of gender, based on male genitalia and socialisation, exempting morality from this analysis entirely. However, the greatest misconception about 'essentialist' vs. 'constructivist' debates between cissexuals and transsexuals is the idea that cissexuals draw on biological essentialism and that transsexuals draw on social constructionism to explain or defend their moral positions on gendered 'truth'. The conflation of cissexual/essential and transsexual/constructivist is flawed because the arguments made on either side do not reflect this clear dichotomy. For example, a cissexual person may reject the legitimacy of a pre-operative transsexual woman by the logic that 'women do not have male genitalia'. Post-surgery, however, the rationale to defend the cissexual position switches to 'women do not undergo male socialisation'. Cissexuals may concede that gender socialisation is based on birth sex and that this is in and of itself a social construction. Conversely, because gender and sex matching is 'typical' for human development, it is easily naturalised. In other words, cissexuals often essentialise social construction to the point that socialisation ironically trumps biological sex. This is because the sexed body in and of itself commits no moral offence, nor is the sexed body particularly morally virtuous. It is the gender-socialised 'owner' of such bodies who subjects the body to interactive sociality, and who holds the moral responsibility of what happens to it. When cissexuals claim that transsexual women are not 'really' women, they are not referring to the sexed body per se, but the distinctly masculine socialisation process the sexed body has undergone (Vernon 2012).

Transsexuals may align theoretically with academic work that posits gender as a social construction, but few would reiterate its core principle to claim that they are 'doing gender', emphasising its intended artifice. And yet, transsexual women do draw on gender as socially constructed because this confirms that although they were raised as men, their socialisation did not take because they have always had an innate sense of gender. Indeed, the argument most transsexual women make is essentialising in that there is a deeply internal and persistent sense that they have always been female. Many do not outright reject the gender binary, nor do they have strong oppositions to the world being divided into male and female as 'natural' as they wish to fit themselves into it. What is problematic in this context, however, is more about the social construction of nature because cissexual gender identities are empirically no more or less 'natural' or 'true' than transsexual gender identities. But what is truly profound here is that transsexuals do not have to reject or adopt either theory to make the moral point of having 'true selves', speaking quite directly to Zigon's notion that morality falls indeed 'within a range of possibilities' (2009: 251). Therefore, cultural debates about essential vs. constructivist perspectives of gender are not just anthropological, but distinctly moral concerns because dominant ciscentric moral models deny that 'true selves' can exist in gendered bodies which have distinctly social and moral histories. Yet these moral models cannot be developed based on a clear distinction of gender as essential or constructed.

Conclusion

Sharpe's encouragement of the investigation of 'how law constructs truth around the facts it demands be disclosed' (2012: 35) is a fitting analogue to how ciscentric morality constructs a particular form of truth around transsexual identities in disclosure contexts. Through the mixed disclosure models of social geographies of knowledge and a language of exclusion, a functional morality emerges: the ciscentric right to know functions as the right to determine (the subjectivity of others), while the transcentric right not to make known functions as the right to self-determine. While my intention in this chapter is to deconstruct and complicate disclosure as a moral concern of transsexual women, I have tried to frame my analysis around anthropological theories of morality whereby majority or hegemonic moral models can be unbalanced by minority claims to moral personhood, so challenging the social consensus.

Zigon's moral 'range of possibilities' resonates in both theory and application. Precisely because the core moral values expressed in cultural practices which distinguish truth from deception are taken-for-granted in everyday worlds, cissexuals remain invested in gender boundaries and the retention of morally sanctioned labelling power. Adverse reactions to transsexuals claiming a subjective sense of gender but rejecting, or modifying, their transsexual life trajectories therefore are directed towards the violation of the social consensus on truth, not social violation of gender norms.

In this chapter, my argument has thus diverged from how essentialist perspectives construct gender in hegemonic ways, to how morality constructs its objects of truth in transsexual disclosure contexts. I concede that the latter is a broader analytical insight about the former, but the difference I argue illuminates the meaning of disclosure as a revelation of truth grounded in shared understanding. All subjective gender experiences are of 'true selves', but only when morality is articulated in disclosure contexts does it become clear how one moral personhood is constructed as more virtuous than another. Thus, transsexual women's strategies of disclosure as moral concerns show that social geographies of knowledge and a language of exclusion navigate around common moral understandings of honesty by yielding to ciscentric concepts of truth while resisting accusations of 'untruthful' presentations of the self. While ciscentric moral models continue to command legal, medical, and institutional power to determine 'true selves', transcentric moral models continue to fight for a moral legitimacy that challenges the social and collaborative foundations and practices of moral consensus in everyday life.

Acknowledgements

I would like to thank Dr Linda Garro, Dr Oscar Gil Garcia and Dr Jarrett Zigon for reading and providing helpful comments for this chapter.

Notes

1 My 2010 dissertation research on the social efficacy of biomedical intervention focused on the social capital transsexual women expected to gain from undergoing genital reassignment surgery (GRS). I spent a year in Trinidad, Colorado, conducting participant observation with fifty transsexual women who had come to Trinidad to undergo surgery with Dr Marci Bowers. I had the unique opportunity to live in a recovery house for GRS patients which provided me with critical insights into transsexual women's perspectives, not only on the expected social efficacy of the surgery, but also on how they negotiated disclosure about their differently gendered past.

2 Stealth denotes the undetected passing as the opposite gender evident in the disconnection from all contexts which could 'out' a person, as much as possible.

3 The only incidents where the stealth model would have been questioned would most likely have come from within the early gay men's movement that pre-dates the era and idea of being openly trans. More importantly, going 'stealth' was generally a clinical requirement or prerequisite to obtaining hormonal or surgical treatment for transsexuals presenting to medical authorities at the time because being openly or visibly trans would have put into question the sincerity or authenticity of the claim of 'really' being a woman/man. This would also have been discrediting to the medical practitioners who were early supporters of transsexuals, validating transsexuals' claims to the scrutinising public.

4 See Sandy Stone's 1991 'Postranssexual Manifesto', urging transsexuals to come out and assert political legitimacy as transsexuals.

5 See Mason-Schrock 1996 on transsexuals' notion of the 'true self'.

6 See Garfinkel 1967 on what constitutes the 'essentialist' position of sex and gender.

7 'Trans-panic' describes the alleged unaccountability of interpersonal violence committed upon discovery of a transsexual's genitalia by cissexuals. But it could also apply to the discovery of a transsexual person's differently gendered history generally, and need not focus on genitalia or the transsexual body alone.

8 Although Sharpe is writing about the legal situation of transsexuals in the UK and Europe, US laws generally follow similar ideas about non-disclosure constituting perceived 'harm' to cissexuals in sexual or marital relationships with transsexuals.

9 Many partners of transsexuals face the same problem of constantly having to explain their relationship to others, if, for example, their currently female partner is also the father of their children.

9 HIV disclosure

Practices, knowledges and ethics

Corinne Squire

HIV disclosure is a technology that allows for treatment, and encourages the development of supportive social bonds, HIV subjectivities, and HIV citizenship and activism. HIV disclosure is also, though, related to criminalisation, to contact tracing and to the stigmatisation and isolation of many people living with the virus. In this chapter, I explore HIV disclosure practices in relation to what is disclosed, who discloses to whom, in what circumstances, and by what means. I consider how these factors relate to stigmatisation or acceptance; isolation or inclusion; disbelief, minimisation or affirmation; and 'responsibilisation', criminalisation and activism. I also examine the relationship between disclosure and knowledge, since HIV knowledge is often uncertain or tied into networks of fears and hopes that may seem irrational and abjectifying. Lastly, I look at disclosure as a required moral narrative for subjects, undermined by both the impossibility of disclosing everything and the ambiguity of told secrets.

Disclosure is a contemporary technology that contributes to medical, social, political and personal governmentalities, that is, to the intersecting practices through which local, national and international organisations produce and regulate subjects and citizens (Foucault 1991). As illustrated in the first chapter of this volume, it has many different realms of operation. In politics, it involves the making public of personal emotional, economic or social interests. In financial services, it requires the making known of personal economic interests. In government, the military and the police, it necessitates making public information about weapons and security when this information is asked for and when the state judges it historically and politically safe to do so. In paid employment, disclosure entails statements about personal, emotional, economic and, in the case of research and development, knowledge interests. In health, it connotes the conveyance of information about personal health, either to those who might reasonably be expected to have interests in it, such as family members, relationship partners, employers and health insurers, or to a more general public. In social life, disclosure often entails making explicit conditions that are unmarked but stigmatised, such as poverty, mental illness, sexual and gender diversity, illegal drug use or criminal convictions.

Disclosure is a particularly modern, even late-modern, technology. It comprises, generally, the transmission of knowledge from a realm understood as private, often personal, to one conceptualised as public. In certain circumstances, this process could be dangerous or unpleasant for the discloser or for others connected to the knowledge. It separates individual subjects from public life, while at the same time turning the personal into a perpetual object of public discussion. Citizenship becomes reduced to a private selfhood whose revelation constitutes the public realm (Rose 1990). Disclosure also involves the dissemination of knowledge, a modern currency, the acquisition of which, like disclosure itself, is never complete. Moreover, knowledge is very often that of a socially transgressive past or present. The contemporary ties between public knowledge, self-knowledge and ethics appear particularly clear in disclosure technologies. Subjects are called to give an explicit account of themselves in order to enter into socio-ethical citizenships (Butler 2005, MacIntyre 1984). Here self-disclosure is inevitably incomplete, betrayed by the exigencies of language and of a subject which comes to know itself as it speaks itself into existence. It is also part of the language and knowledge of power within which ethics sits (Foucault 1997, Friedman and Squire 1998).

Disclosure also has many earlier precedents: in Christian confession, for instance (Manderson, this volume); in the continuing cathartic aspects of traditional health and spiritual technologies; and in histories of governmentality that have depended, in Western capitalist states, on making visible subject characteristics in order to allow their monitoring and regulation by state, society and self (Foucault 1975). The condition of HIV is frequently lived with alongside stigmatisation, 'othering' and secrecy (Joffe 2006), and the dangers of revelation are often extremely clear. HIV therefore instantiates the complexities of disclosure in the case of health.

Knowledge, practices and ethics

HIV is a virus transmitted, with some difficulty, via certain human body fluids. HIV disclosure concerns another kind of transmission – that of knowledge – usually in relation to HIV status, although also whether someone has been tested, is on treatment or is ill. These disclosures can have medical, legal and social implications.

Disclosure in general passes knowledge, usually about persons – oneself or others – from one person to another. Knowledge cannot be understood adequately, however, if it is treated as unproblematically transmissible. Knowledge transmission, like HIV transmission, is complicated, affected by the state of what is being transmitted, who is transmitting it and who is receiving it.

One way to approach these complexities is to consider whether disclosure is simply transitive, and whether it always has an indirect object, the object disclosed to. When people describe disclosing their HIV status, they sometimes simply say, 'I disclosed': the object is left implicit. This omission could be treated as indicative of broader difficulties of saying everything about HIV. Again, people describing their disclosure sometimes include but sometimes exclude an indirect object in the dative case: the person, people or organisation disclosed to. Of course, disclosure always does have such an object or objects: it is a dialogic process. However, the frequent omission of the indirect object also indicates wider problems of pinning down who is being disclosed to, and whether the disclosure has been received. In the light of these difficulties, it might be easier to view disclosing not merely as a verb signifying an activity, but also as a metaphor for a particular set of personal, social and institutional practices. In relation to HIV, for instance, 'I disclosed', regardless of its object and indirect object, often suggests personal openness. At times, it can have revelatory connotations that seem to provide a heavily moralised template for the passing on of knowledge that is rather different from straightforward knowledge transmission. Moreover, the knowledge that comes from HIV disclosure is frequently not what might be expected. More generally than disclosure, then, in this chapter I am concerned with practices, particularly practices of knowledge around HIV. I shall, like Manderson (this volume), move my discussion from practices, through knowledge, to ethics.

Like other illnesses, HIV does not just exist as a medical condition, but as a set of past, present, future and imagined, cultural, social and ethical practices. For this reason, HIV disclosure is never just about HIV or disclosure; it is a particular kind of event, one that varies according to context (Iwelunmor et al. 2010). Stigmatisation and discrimination around the condition mean that disclosure has special salience: it has implications for work, relationships, children, sexuality, criminalisation, citizenship, social isolation and interpersonal violence. HIV disclosure has to be treated carefully by disclosers, audiences and those who make policy about it.

Living with HIV is also not fully distinct from other everyday conditions of living. For many people, HIV disclosure is a regular part of daily life; for many more, a frequent topic of discussion or thought. This applies particularly where HIV is a high-prevalence condition, especially in sub-Saharan Africa; in specific communities, for instance, some city and rural communities in the USA, particularly for Latino and African Americans; among African migrants in high-income countries; and among gay men in countries at many income levels. In London, approximately one in twelve gay men is estimated to be HIV positive (Health Protection Agency 2012). Within such high-prevalence situations, HIV's hiding and disclosure within family, friendship and work networks are routine concerns. HIV is an everyday secret, like other health or socio-moral conditions, such as TB, cancer, syphilis, mental illness, illegitimacy or criminality.

The contemporary extension of HIV treatment access to 10 million of the 34 million people living with HIV, over 50% of those who need it (UNAIDS 2012), and the possibility and anticipation of treatment for others (Davis and Squire 2010), has contributed to resituating HIV and its disclosure as everyday. It has also changed the knowledge on which HIV disclosure trades, resituating HIV positivity as a 'long-term condition' (Health Protection Agency 2011) rather than a fatal illness. Ethically, too, the possibility of HIV treatment in the contemporary era has reframed HIV disclosure as easier, a moral call now less likely to involve personal and social suffering, and as less necessary and more contested, because, if treatment has lowered viral load to undetectable levels, HIV transmission risk is low even if condoms are not used (Cohen et al. 2011).

(Not) researching disclosure

In this chapter, I draw on a 2011 study of HIV support in the UK, which included forty-seven interviews (50% gay or bisexual men, 25% heterosexual men, 25% women). The interviews were not about disclosure, but they contained extensive material on disclosure (see also Squire 2013). Moreover, taking part in an interview explicitly about HIV is already a kind of disclosure, to the interviewer and to oneself. In this way, the study implicitly presupposes disclosure as one of its interests.

Most interviewees were taking antiretroviral medication. Although they were doing well by the markers of CD4 count and low viral load, most had moderate to severe health problems. Disclosing their HIV status was therefore not the disclosure of an unproblematic, well-treated health condition: this is probably a minority experience (National AIDS Trust 2011). Around one-third of the interviewees participated in prior rounds of the study, dating from 2001 and in some cases from 1997 or 1993 (see Squire 1999, 2003, 2006). The study therefore included a relatively large number of participants aged over 50 and who had considerable psychosocial and illness experience of living with HIV before the advent of anti-retroviral treatment in the UK in 1996. Their perspectives on disclosure were strongly affected by these histories of HIV as a fatal, untreatable condition, which for ex-IV drug users and gay men, killed large numbers of lovers and friends. In addition, around one-third of study participants were African-origin migrants, for whom disclosure had a doubled history within both the UK and their home countries. In sub-Saharan Africa, treatment has only been available to the majority who need it since 2011, and prevalence of infection is much higher than in the UK. Hence, HIV disclosure has until very recently been the disclosure of a fatal condition affecting all families.

In this study, some participants were recruited by chain sampling. These included interviewees whose difficulties with living with and disclosing HIV were intense, and, on the other hand, interviewees for whom HIV appeared to be simply one of many of the conditions of their life, about which they were freely disclosing. Most participants, however, volunteered via websites and NGOs. Both people at ease with living with HIV and those who have strong dis-ease with the condition are unlikely to take part through these mechanisms, unless re-contacted from earlier study rounds. Even in this case, some participants from earlier rounds fell into these categories. One woman, first interviewed a decade ago, described herself as too beset with illness, only partly HIV-related, to want to participate again. Another prior participant who had moved away from her earlier HIV-related work said she did not want to spend time on a condition that was now a minor part of her life. In such instances, HIV has a powerful valency that people may not want to revisit via the disclosures involved in interviews. People more recently diagnosed may have decided not to participate in the study because HIV was an unremarkable, well-treated and fully accepted part of their lives. However, given the stories of stigmatisation and isolation told by recently diagnosed people who volunteered for this interview round, the disclosures required in interviews may have seemed too overwhelming for some. Participants in this round can thus be inferred to include those who recognised some difficulties around living with HIV, but who were able also to countenance giving the disclosing self-accounts that interviews ask for.

The study involved practices or enactments of disclosure, within the interview themes of support, and within the self-story that such interviews generate (Riessman 2008). Interviews can be described as specific kinds of narratives, but they can also usefully be thought of, in relation to disclosure, as hybridising talk with friends; consultations with consultants; counselling sessions; assessments with professionals; and diaristic or autobiographical forms, or 'talking to oneself' (see, for instance, Kvale 2008). Interview disclosure draws on all these genres as well as on the disclosure genre produced by the researcher's and the research participant's understandings of research.

I used narrative analysis to address the interview materials, understanding 'narrative', broadly, as involving meaningful movements or sequences of symbols that build up meaning (Squire 2012, see also Andrews et al. 2013). I adopted this approach for a number of reasons. First, people often talk about disclosure via anecdotes or stories of specific events, or via 'habitual narratives' that generalise what often happens to themselves or others. Second, within semi-structured interviews, prolonged, fragmented and complicated stories of HIV disclosure often developed across the course of the interviews, moving from well-worn tales of how disclosure does or does not work, towards more ambiguous narrative endings, adding complexity to disclosure. Third, a second etymological root of 'narrative' lies in knowledge itself: stories are means of telling but also of working towards or through knowledge. Treating the interview material as narrative alerts its readers to its active struggles for and with knowledge.

Disclosure practices and knowledge

Disclosure of knowledge about HIV status involves a set of particular practices, but it is also part of a constellation of life practices. Sometimes it is connected to technologies of external governance, sometimes to technologies of more intimate interpersonal or self-governance. Sometimes its practices are complex and hard to trace. In what follows, I outline some of these practices and their ambiguities as they emerged in the research.

Disclosure and governmentality

Within medical and social services, HIV disclosure is often planned and implemented by degrees on the basis of 'need to know', a term prevalent in social work discourse particularly, and taken over from military use (see also Vernon, this volume). Those who 'need to know' are usually identified as those closest to the HIV-positive person, most intimately concerned with their care and with transmission-risk situations. Often, these people are advised or even required to know, particularly where ART (antiretroviral treatment) is new and unfamiliar, where there may be bad reactions or side-effects, or a need for other care, or where they may be at HIV risk themselves. Professionals such as GPs, dentists and chiropodists may not be required to know but may be thought to benefit from knowing. Yet, even on this need-to-know basis, disclosure is understood to be potentially problematic: family, friends and partners may reject you, professionals may not want to treat you. Quentin, a black African migrant living in London, in his forties, diagnosed in 1995, had, like a number of other interviewees, found it very difficult to get a dentist who seemed comfortable treating HIV positive patients. He was also having considerable problems with his medication, which exacerbated his concerns about disclosing to his GP:

> If you have problems to get GP, some practice they don't have dentist and sometimes teeth, dentist, dentist is very hard. And this how you become scared, I have to disclose as you for example go to/mhm/doctor or dentist. This is when you say 'I have to disclose', for example when you go to dentist you have to disclose as far as I know some colleagues or some people the same as my situation they say if you disclose they don't give you appointment. They say maybe they give you longer time, you have to disclose or not because as far as I know some people some might, many, many people they say that to see a doctor take you a long time/mhm/This is our, sometimes at the GP, you describe, you have to disclose because some GPs they don't know about HIV and either they give you medication they don't know/Sure/If sometimes they give you medication, they can't, hah/Can't work/Yeah (laughs) can't work.

Disclosure to professionals is thus presented as necessary for treatment success but sometimes also leads to rejection or loss of confidentiality: 'Sometimes you can see yourself with a red mark' (on the GP file), another interviewee, Queenie, a woman of African origin in her fifties, said.

Interviewees also registered requirements to disclose to lawyers and others dealing with asylum cases, and to those who needed to know because of the possibility of the criminalisation of HIV transmission, including lawyers and, most problematically, sexual partners. Many interviewees had developed disclosure strategies to address this latter issue, such as immediate disclosure to people who interested them sexually, or serosorting online or via print ads or particular social venues (see Davis and Flowers, this volume). However, fears about the criminalisation of non-disclosure in intimate relationships and the disclosing potential of condoms themselves prevented some interviewees, such as Quentin, from having relationships at all:

> And, hah, about the social lifestyle, to have partner (stammers) to have but or to have, this is another issue because you have to stick with sometime with the same situation. Otherwise it affects the law or how even when you have sex outside, you have to be conscience about that or if you have to use condoms, and sometimes when you meet [with] those condom and so on and so, they suspect you.

Disclosure was also reported as planned and performed, in relation to known protection policies at work and their alleged failures, with varying outcomes: from full disclosure working well across diverse work situations, to disclosure on employment applications resulting in failure.

Disclosure of HIV status is never really freely provided. It is always part of a contract in which things such as services, citizenship, relationships or personhood are given back. However, the neoliberal regulation of individual biomedical HIV subjects via disclosure-based 'technologies of subjectivity' (Ong 2006: 6, Rose 2007) had reached new heights when I undertook the interviews in 2011, compared, for instance, with the interviews in 2001. People brought me letters declaring their status officially, lest I not believe them. It appeared that HIV disclosure was popularly understood as a form of currency for people with few resources, and so needed legitimation. A more prevalent understanding of disclosure technologies for HIV positive people, however, was as very strongly 'responsibilising', as Quentin described, again in relation to medical professionals, who, he explained, had the right to know and even not to treat:

> You are worried if you reveal this disclosure, you may be, you say I prefer not to tell them and you are feeling you have to tell them, in order to protect them for me because sometimes it takes the opposite, better when they know you[r status] and may not treat you, I don't know, fairly or but that is why you should give them knowledge or lack of knowledge or information about them, because some(thing) is affecting us, them also.

In such narrative progressions, the governance of HIV by disclosure becomes internally, intimately felt and enacted: 'If some(thing) is affecting us, them also.'

Disclosure and intimate governance

At more intimate levels of self-regulation, HIV disclosure is a practice in relation to other HIV practices. For instance, it is planned in relation to how family members have reacted to prior experiences of HIV among people close to them, to what the partner thinks and says about condoms, to how friends discuss HIV when it's on the television or on World AIDS Day. In addition, the family's, partners' and friends' rights are not exactly to know HIV status, but to the kind of intimacy involved with this status knowledge, without which something in these relationships would be seen as compromised or inauthentic (Davis and Flowers 2011). So HIV disclosure is also one of a set of connected practices around health, sexuality and reproduction, work and relationships.

Most research participants had plans for when to disclose in intimate relationships, and for when they would disclose to family members. The conditions were usually face-to-face meetings when they were in good health, although sometimes, if participants were generally well, they described plans to disclose only if they were getting ill. Obtaining resources or citizenship status were also often preconditions within stories of planned disclosure, to allow participants to support themselves, not to trouble families, or to leave partners if they reacted negatively.

Sometimes these forms of HIV disclosure are externally regulated, for instance, via contact tracing procedures or health or social welfare professional strictures about who ought to be disclosed to and when, especially in relation to partners, ex-partners and children. Mostly, however, within participants' own narratives, disclosures were positioned within exchanges of emotions, intimacy and care. Queenie described a process of this kind in relation to her pastor. Although her story might seem to be about institutional disclosure, for Queenie, the relationship with the pastor was important:

> Yeah, [the pastor] does [understand about HIV], because he even says 'Don't be shy talking about it, yeah. You can come for counselling, you can talk, even if you are ill in hospital.' Like my pastor Henry, I told him. Yeah, yeah I told him but it took time for me to tell him, yeah. Yeah, I told him /yes/, he really supports me, even when I'm down or ill. Sometimes if he doesn't see me, he calls me, 'Are you OK, do you want someone to come and pray for you or talk to you?' Or even if I'm admitted to hospital he comes. I feel loved. There's no strings attached yeah, which is good. [Short exchange about not/telling congregation

members.] Some people feel like they can't tell the pastor either/Yeah, yeah/. It depends on the relationship, that is why I said with me it took time. I was there in the church studying him, it took time for me, about three years, yeah. Then deep down in my spirit, I said 'Oh yeah, I have to tell him now. I think I have to tell him now.' I was ready, yeah.

This story demonstrates a common form across the interviews in its moves from intimate observation and evaluation, through disclosure, to acceptance and emotional progression. In the later development of this narrative towards a retrospectively given origin in reflexive consideration, 'deep down in my spirit', we can also see the associations between practices of intimate, interpersonal governmentality and self-governance.

Disclosure and self-governmentality

For the narrated self, disclosure may work as a practice that can release or heal. Some participants who described themselves as knowing about HIV and accepting it also described HIV knowledge, kept inside, as 'eating away at them'. As a non-shared secret, it was corrosive. Such interviewees said that a disclosing openness enabled them to become 'fuller' versions of themselves, an approach that built on the processes of working through HIV acceptance through what might be called disclosure to oneself. Disclosure was thus articulated as part of a more general self-actualisation happening through the 'testing' route of HIV.

This is a relatively neutral description of self-disclosure and governmentality, marking the general psychologising of social lives (Rose 1990). From it, we might understand the processes in operation as restricting possibility within research participants' lives. Such processes could be seen as a technology of what MacIntyre (1984) describes as 'emotivism', which reduces understandings of all social and political relations to personal emotions sequestered from full public comprehension but ciphered, regulated and exchanged as a general currency. Within contemporary neoliberalism, the coding and management of subjectivities has become ferociously technical (Elliott 2013, Ong 2006). Nguyen (2010), for example, has described how international NGOs, especially in low-income situations, baldly require a particular form of HIV subject – self-aware, articulate and emotionally resolved – if they are to provide treatment.

However, technologies of governmentality are not homogeneous in character. They can be part of progressive and activist framings of the pandemic. In stories of living with HIV, for example, 'I disclosed to her/him' is often a testifying, ethically loaded moment. Such stories can expand the minimalised nature of neoliberal HIV subjects and the people around them because, within them, disclosure 'tests' oneself and the other person ethically. Something is, after struggle, confessed. As with all confessions, this one requires something of the person to whom confession is made, as well as of the person confessing. Disclosure is a dialogue, a disclosure *to* someone, not a transmission, a disclosure *of* something. Disclosure therefore makes a moral call as well as providing knowledge.

This self-technology is frequently tied into more collective articulations of HIV acceptance and activism. Disclosure is positioned in many HIV advocacy and activism contexts as a condition of action, a way of claiming space as a political biomedical subject, using but also subverting the language of health and human rights (Mbali 2005, Robins 2009, Rose 2007). Disclosure thus becomes a part of a political technology of 'speaking out', similar to South American traditions of *testimonio* (Beverley 2004) against state violence, drawing on but not reducible to religious testimony. Where this politics of disclosure is entirely absent, one can often see real political difficulties. The fragmented and isolated situation of HIV-positive people in Serbia and Montenegro, with no one publically speaking out as and for people living with HIV, illustrates this well (Bernays et al. 2007). However, the contemporary invisibility of the HIV epidemic in the UK, frequently commented on by interviewees, offers a similar if better-resourced picture. One interviewee commented on the negative reactions, even ridicule, he had encountered online when he suggested a UK movement to wear 'HIV positive' T shirts of the 'trademark' kind that played a key symbolic role for many South Africans in owning the epidemic both personally and socially (e.g. Heywood 2009: 19). With a more positive outcome, Queenie described her contested but finally successful attempts to affirm her own HIV status in order to testify to and help others. These attempts were themselves enabled by a micro-social world of intimate disclosures between friends and within support groups, and by a framing of disclosure as supported by faith:

> So yeah, you have to be open, yeah, because you want to help this person, yeah. So, you have to be open and share your experiences . . . that way you will help /yeah/ and after then you can still talk on the phone if it's possible, yeah. You can say 'how are you doing, any challenges, any problems?' You know, you try to refer to what I did; to me, I did this and this; try this one, try this one, yeah . . . This [HIV positive] friend [of my sister] took me to a support group. But I was shy to go there. I said 'oh they will look at me; they will point fingers at me'. He said 'no', he said 'look at me, I am positive'. And when I went in there, I saw happy faces. Then, I was asking, and she said 'no, everybody in here is HIV positive'. 'So do you think I will be like that one or that one?' I said, 'Look they are (feeling) strong and beautiful'. She said 'you will, you will', but yeah. So, I remember that day, the first day, it really empowered me, yeah. From then, I kept on going and going, as well, yeah. And my religion helped as well, yeah, my religion.

The complexities of HIV disclosure practices

Disclosure practices are not always as simple as they may seem. A disclosing HIV positive subject may have to negotiate his or her status as an HIV-positive citizen at work, where it may have implications on types of activity and times of absence; in relationships, where it may affect sexual and reproductive practices, types of emotional connection, economic support and interpersonal violence; and in the family and among friends, where a person may be accepted like any other, or seen as a vulnerable child, a compromised parent or a figure of contagion and terror from whom others withdraw.

HIV disclosure involves disclosures about a life and not just an HIV status. It may make sense of or cascade into knowledge about other medical issues, mental health issues, relationships, children and bereavements. HIV disclosure for an asylum seeker in the UK, for instance, was also sometimes a disclosure about the necessity of leaving one's children in a country of origin with poor treatment access, and the impossibility of returning to them without citizenship status or money. For a person in this situation, the story of their children was often the most important one they told about HIV. Other interviewees, such as Quentin, told stories of stigmatisation and isolation, of 'dying twice' (Campbell et al. 2007), which were, for them, the most significant aspects of HIV disclosure.

Even where treatment is accessible and successful, and friends are supportive, HIV disclosure may be constituted as an equation between life and 'being HIV' (see Davis and Flowers, this volume), rather than simply as a transmission of status knowledge. Sean, a man in his early thirties, characterising himself and his twenty-something boyfriend as HIV positive, presented this status as the entirety of their lives. They were relatively recently diagnosed, and both had had considerable problems with HIV-related illness and with ART side-effects. They were not, Sean said, 'living with HIV'; they *were* HIV.

HIV disclosure can, vicariously, disclose something about other people's lives, and hence disclosure does not affect just one person. If a person discloses their positive status, their whole family may experience associational shame. Queenie's disclosure of her diagnosis told her children, who ranged from primary age to young adulthood, something quite definite, not just about their late father's HIV status but also about his character:

> My children they were very angry, yeah, they were very angry; especially, because they were accusing their father/The older children? /All of them, yeah. As soon as I had told them, they accused him because their Dad passed in 1997 . . . So, when he died, he died when we were separated about two years ago, two years when he died. But they knew, because of the way he died. But with myself, I didn't know, because it was two years after I had left him . . . So they were accusing their Dad, yeah, they were very angry. And, I ended up, I said 'you know, there's

no point because he's dead now, and I'm still alive. You just have to concentrate, erm, to concentrate, help me to pull through. And you, yourself as well, yeah, we have to work at this together; because if (you) are down and angry, it affects me as well, and I will deteriorate as well.' Now, they are fine.

HIV disclosure also works by metaphor or metonymy to disclose other socially stereotyped aspects of self: sexuality, sexual history, children, moral personhood. The enormous rhetorical freight HIV drags around with it was early and well documented (Crimp 1988, Sontag 1989, Treichler 1999, Watney 1994). The power of these associations is indexed by the near inevitability that disclosure is followed by questions not just about health, but also ethically weighted issues about mode of infection and practices of containment.

The associations commonly attached to HIV disclosure in the UK are with homosexuality and bisexuality; sexual irresponsibility or transgression, for instance, sex outside a primary relationship; sex work; sex with people of African origin, bisexual or homosexual men; or intravenous drug use or sex with someone who uses drugs. For people recently diagnosed, HIV disclosure may also suggest credulity, carelessness or mental health problems. Many interviewees disclosed their status during interviews in ways that told 'how I got it' while also exempting them from such charges. One man in his twenties, for example, started the interview with the story of 'my cheating ex'; another man in his thirties described an earlier time of depression and intensive drug use. Queenie positioned the time and place where she likely became HIV positive as one when little was known about HIV. Ora, a white British woman in her thirties, emphasised, through a long account of the failure to diagnose her illnesses as HIV-related, her failure to fit her own and others' HIV risk profile, since she had not had sexual experiences or partners connected to the epidemic.

HIV disclosure can also *happen* indirectly, by association. These disclosures are manifold: medications in the bathroom or a bag; new habits of cooking and eating healthy foods; multivitamins in the house; keeping ART-related regular hours; less partying, drinking or doing drugs; continuing single status; new friendships with HIV positive people; work with HIV organisations; use of particular clinics or other services associated with HIV; conversations about HIV; the deaths or HIV-linked illnesses of partners, ex-partners and children; not breastfeeding; having a Caesarian section; having pneumonia, TB, meningitis, rashes, weight loss, shingles, herpes or 'cancer'; putting 'rather not say' on a Gaydar profile under 'HIV status'; not using condoms; using condoms; or simply displaying, as Quentin noted, a new mood that your friends notice:

Even some people they start to ask me, 'Your skill is changed, you are not happy, you took', sometime (my friend) he ask me 'Why you took a lot of tabs'. I say this is because I have got – sometime I say, I have to lie. 'Yah, no, no! I have got some problem with my kidney or my (sugar) and the doctor', all those things.

This cloud of associational possibilities is not surprising, given HIV's own powerful symbolic weight. However, it compounds the nebulousness of disclosure practices, since not only what is disclosed, but also how disclosure happens, becomes diffuse, attached to the fearful recruitment of many different physical, biomedical, psychological and social signs.

The refusal to disclose is itself a disclosure practice. In many contexts, people work effectively as HIV activists without declaring their HIV status. Arguments around political or community solidarity can turn a disclosure requirement into something divisive, or frame it as an external demand for inappropriate and possibly dangerous openness (Nguyen 2010). The responsibilisation of the HIV-positive person to speak out could be seen as a parallel to criminalisation, removing responsibility from seronegative others. A number of interviewees narrated their own disclosure refusals in this way. In such accounts, non-disclosure was part of their practices of protecting or owning HIV knowledge themselves, and also a way of reframing that knowledge. Robert, for example, a white British man in his forties, narrated this potentially empowering, though sometimes highly stigmatising, non-disclosure as operating within HIV discourse, irrespective of status:

> I was treated really badly by someone, I hadn't disclosed my status, but didn't do anything risky, and he made me feel like shit, and what was really great was a friend of mine who works in [HIV organisation] I phoned him up because he's a wise old sage, 'I feel like crap', he said, like, 'Tell him to fuck off', he said, 'if he's so concerned about staying negative he should have said "I'm negative", blah blah blah, from the outset.' He said, 'I'm fed up with', he's negative himself, my friend, 'I'm fed up with these people expecting a positive person to disclose. If they're so desperate to stay negative then they should do it.'

When successfully taking ART, there may be little reason, in relation to transmission, for a person who knows they are HIV positive and who is using condoms to disclose. Their risk of transmitting HIV, even if they do not use condoms, is low (Cohen et al. 2011). The risk of someone becoming infected by having sex with someone who cannot disclose because they are not tested and who is more infectious because not treated, is much higher; in the UK, 20–25% of those who are HIV positive do not know their status (Health Protection Agency 2012). At times, interviewees articulated this new aspect of medical technology alongside their rejection of the responsibilisation of HIV-positive people for disclosure. However, interviewees taking ART, mostly aware of their own low transmission risk, were also deeply responsibilised and at times abjectified by their own non-disclosures, as Robert's repeatedly conveyed: 'he made me feel like crap . . . I feel like shit'.

The failure of HIV knowledge among those who have not tested, or who have tested and not collected their test results, points to one absolute barrier to disclosure. In addition, some interviewees told stories about earlier suspecting their status, but not knowing for sure, or of disbelieving the test. Moreover, HIV disclosure is always disclosure of a particular knowledge of HIV; you may not disclose because you understand HIV as fatal; or as something that has killed many other family members; or as a condition that leads to social exile; or as a condition whose infectiousness, once treated, is medically unlikely but personally frightening.

Disclosure and ethics

As mentioned, disclosure is a socio-ethical imperative. Subjects have to give accounts of who they are and what they do in order to take up a social place. But, in such an account, the person must speak from a position of knowledge and morality that they do not fully occupy, glossing over moral complexities and fixing themselves within an ultimately fluid language, as Butler (2005), following Lacan, notes. It is especially difficult to achieve this moral, disclosing, but necessarily tenuous self-account when one's position is also destabilised by HIV's physical seriousness, stigmatisation and uncertainties.

Treatment may seem to ease the moral ambiguities around HIV, but HIV's treatment-driven normalisation can also drive such ambiguities underground. Within the UK HIV support study, participants who were HIV positive, healthy and well supported often asserted this condition as the current, normalised state of HIV (Squire 2013). At the same time, almost all noted other, more difficult states of living with HIV, which they had heard about, seen or experienced themselves in the past, and which can still happen, even with new drugs taken early. Sometimes they described these states in a still-normalised, medicalised way, as a form of accelerated ageing. At other times, they told more clearly pessimistic stories, for instance, of HIV-associated cancers, neuropathy, dementia, perhaps a chosen death, other feared and unknown HIV-related conditions, and stigmatisation and social exclusion. Current neoliberal restructurings and withdrawals of services intensify these subtextual negative knowledges. Even with improved services, however, such knowledges would likely continue unless HIV became much more medically manageable and socially destigmatised. Presently, they tend to make disclosure practices more complex, blurring what it means to disclose HIV status, and positioning such disclosure as more heterogeneous than a straightforward understanding of HIV as treatable and treated would suggest.

Disclosure reveals things kept secret, but secrets can never be fully revealed, and some things about HIV remain secret and cannot be shared or revealed (Derrida 2001). HIV status disclosure does not tell everything, yet it also tells too much. Disclosing can expose and depersonalise someone, taking things away from them. It gives them the name of the virus and substitutes that for their own name, their own person, even for themselves: 'I am HIV.'

Derrida (2001) suggests that the condition of ethics is for people to be respected and acknowledged without having to tell everything – to be able to have a secret. Ethics requires us to recognise the other without knowing anything – let alone everything – about them. The kinds of proxy HIV disclosures discussed above, via, for instance, lifestyle changes, instantiate the proxy-ness of all HIV disclosures. Disclosure never tells us everything about living with serious, potentially fatal illness, and the uncertainties of it, nor about the possibilities of its limited effects, of being able to live well and healthily. The materiality of the condition, inaccessible to disclosure practices – physical illnesses and fluctuations, daily drug regimes, the experienced effects of both, mental states of depression, anxiety and stress, as well as the healthy and unremarkable daily lives of many HIV positive people – index this incompleteness. This materiality, registered in the many fragmented and sometimes contradictory particularities of participants' stories, marks the inevitable failures of disclosure and the secreted persistence of things that cannot really be revealed.

Many activists argue that disclosure needs to be rethought for the new context of HIV as a long-term, perhaps soon a curable, condition. HIV transmission risk can now be reduced prophylactically, decreased by effective treatment, and removed in some cases by very early treatment. In this situation, the epidemic may best be addressed by focusing on living with HIV in the context of community and relationships, safety and prosperity, health and happiness, rather than in the context of disclosure and its associated fear. For some, though, a focus on 'status', to which disclosure is tied, can be a hindrance. HIV disclosure should rather become part – a rather minor part – of a set of practices of a non-regulatory kind. It might even become irrelevant. These framings move either towards openness or towards the irrelevance of openness as a political strategy. In both cases, the framings position HIV knowledge and HIV's relations to subjecthood in a way that does not just secrete this knowledge in the bodies of the HIV positive, ready to be disclosed, but that moves it out into the HIV-affected world, taking it to every citizen, as the wearing of 'HIV positive' T shirts does. This critical disclosure perspective is not yet the place from which all the participants in the HIV support study seemed to be speaking. But it was certainly a position that they often tried to occupy.

10 Contours of truth

Mark Davis and Lenore Manderson

Disclosure permeates social existence. As the authors contributing to this volume show, in different ways, we make our identities and our connections with others by sharing life stories, experiences and innermost desires. Some tellings are prosaic; others are transformative. Some tellings are resisted, even passed over or implied; others are sought out, rehearsed, cultivated and, at times, staged. Disclosures can happen just once or may be repeated, changed like any narrative to fit the content and the moment. Although disclosure conceptually implies intentionality, some disclosures occur unexpectedly, in ways that strip the person of agency. Other disclosures are chosen and timed; others are required. Disclosure reveals the person who tells, but it also asks something of the person or persons who receive the information.

Disclosure is not particular to health or medical care, although the chapters in this volume focus on the intricacies of disclosure in and around health and illness. Even so, we have explored the playing-out of disclosure in diverse settings and circumstances, with cases and analyses chosen diversely from family life of the urban poor in India, online disclosure of chlamydia in the metropoles of the global North, and the management of HIV identities in families, churches and villages in Africa. In the chapters in this volume, contributing authors have addressed depression and other serious mental illnesses, Huntington's disease, narcolepsy and sex re-assignment. In writing about these different examples and their distinctive social contours, they have posed questions of disclosure as experience, as practice and as an expression of the knowledge economy. And they have examined disclosure for its ramifications in the generation of social science knowledge, given its resonance with performative storytelling and in the ethics of intersubjectivity in research.

In bringing together this collection, we have sought out nuanced understandings of disclosure where, in general, it has had a taken-for-granted status in discourse on health and medicine. In taking this approach, we have resisted the inclination to define and narrow down disclosure; resisted the temptation to make it an object of scrutiny amenable to deductive analysis and so to be measured in association with social characteristics. We have, for example, eschewed the idea that the disclosure of mental illness might result in better prognoses for individuals: we do not – collectively and individually – take the view that disclosure is necessarily a 'good' thing, or that the outcome of disclosure is closure and so resolution. Instead, avoiding the premature reduction of disclosure and the exclusion of related practices, we have tried to open up our understanding of disclosure, empirically and philosophically, so as to build theory and insight about it. In the process, in the analyses presented in the contributory chapters in this volume, we have noted how what we have learned of disclosure might articulate with other domains of life where disclosure is implicated. Sexuality, gender, parenthood, family, community, belief, ethical engagement and responsible citizenship are all implicated in the case studies and conceptual framings of health and illness disclosure in this volume. These contact points between health and illness disclosure and other forms of disclosure – and the wider consideration of truth telling and confession – seem particularly salient given the gathering importance of biotechnology and biological knowledge of social and psychological existence in our social worlds (Clarke et al. 2010).

As the authors of the chapters in this volume have made plain, disclosure is only on occasion overt, singular and discrete. Although the term connotes intentionality and deliberation, if not calculation based on the costs and benefits of exposure, it can be explicit or tacit. Identities are opened to transformation by the assignation and transmission of a biomedical label, and what is often regarded as disclosure in the published literature attends to the impact of diagnosis on individual patients and their psychic life. But this is a narrow reading of the act of disclosure, and the social life that follows from this act. Bodies disclose themselves too, obviating or requiring forms of telling of oneself: weight loss or gain, changes in energy levels, pallor or demeanour – all suggest states open to interpretation, inviting or making redundant the need for spoken disclosure. While we commonly think of disclosure as requiring physical and cognitive alertness and that responsibility to others flows from this, neurological shakiness, sleepiness, gender, looking depressed, can also disclose and/or require an explanation that is a disclosure. Disclosure may also be partial, hinted at or titrated, carefully revealed with wriggle room for its consequences to be deflected or moderated. Intentionality is at stake in disclosure, since it might happen without one's knowledge or despite (or perhaps because of) one's best efforts at avoiding it.

In the contributing chapters, we have illustrated disclosure's complexities, and demonstrated how disclosures are also axiomatically concerned with the circulation of knowledge of one's body, mind and health status and their social effects. To disclose in the first person implies self-subjectification: one takes oneself as a subject of knowledge. In health and medicine this often means making explicit one's diagnosis and its implications for risk to others. In this concluding chapter, we draw together the themes and insights from the contributing chapters, to reflect on how subjectivity, knowledge and truth claims underpin disclosure. Before we do that, however, we map out further the key themes arising from the foregoing analyses. Below, we trace out the theories of self and social relations employed by our authors, pointing out the significance of disclosure in theory of social experience. We also turn to the cross-cutting themes of contexts and strategies of disclosure, as are apparent in the chapters in this volume. We consider disclosure's connections with biography, time and memory, and disclosure's implications for public life, before concluding with some consideration of the implications of the analytical currents of this volume for wider concerns of disclosure, knowledge and truth claims, and their contestations and contradictions.

Disclosure and social theory

Several of our authors have emphasised the experiential aspects of disclosure and so consider how disclosure takes shape, with implications for those who disclose and others in their social worlds. By way of example, we include Kokanovic's and Philip's account of the disclosure narratives of people with mental illness where they spoke of their relationship with doctors, spouses, families and in the workplace; Root's exploration of the accounts of men and women with HIV and the implications of disclosure for one's presence in church and other gatherings; and Vernon's account of the moral imperatives applied to telling the truth of one's gender transitions. These approaches borrow from dramaturgy and Goffman's related notions of stigma management and presentation of self in everyday life (1959, 1963). On this basis, disclosures can be taken to be deeply enmeshed within the management of the social standing of the person who discloses, hence the reworking of disclosures against context, setting and audience. This emphasis on the experience of disclosure resonates with Mead's phenomenology of 'I and me' (Mead 1913), as it does, too, with Freud's id, ego and superego (Freud 1962 [1927]). Disclosure can be taken to be a process of identity formation, the psychological internalisation of what it is believed others see in oneself and extant social requirements regarding one's conduct.

Dramaturgy and psychology, however, are not the only methods by which disclosure can be usefully illuminated. Authors in this volume have drawn on Foucauldian notions of disclosure as a technology of self, and therefore as a mode of self-regulation opened to social norms (Foucault 1988). To disclose is to address, in some way, social norms: the decision to tell of oneself is framed precisely in terms of personal consistency or discordance with normativity. Telling of oneself is a way of making oneself visible in terms that are understood by others in one's social world: the person who discloses sets out the salient facts of the self against conventions of behaviour and belief. This is partly why the disclosures of diagnostic labels or biomedical experiences have such import; they reflect how one might not be the same as others, as marked different or particular. Disclosure of self thus concerns one's difference from a given norm, in relation to the health or another characteristic of the population. The act of disclosure, consequently, reinforces the norm: the point of disclosing (as transgender, as an injecting drug user, as schizophrenic, for instance) is only significant because these particular statuses diverge from mainstream social morality. This framework of disclosure as a statement of divergence draws attention, also, to panopticism, and therefore illustrates how disclosure makes one visible in social relations in particular ways (Foucault 1982).

Following from this, identity signs are manipulated in disclosure. As Davis and Flowers have noted, the fixing and circulation of biomedical signs, as occurs with diagnostic categories presented in online communication, is one way in which one can make oneself visible to others. In this mode of disclosure as visibility, non-verbal signs such as clothes, speech style and so on can also be disclosing. This is, of course, a pedestrian yet politically volatile aspect of everyday life in many settings: a woman who wears a hijab consciously presents herself – discloses herself to a wider, anonymous public – as Muslim.

A number of authors in this volume have drawn on Judith Butler's work (2005), and her use of Foucault and Levinas, among others, to attend to the ways in which the telling of oneself escapes meaning. Not everything about oneself can be recalled and relayed to others. Failed memory, repression and extra-discursive aspects of embodied life all mean that some modes of experience are not amenable to disclosure. Disclosure's partial nature means, therefore, that one of its social effects is to join its interlocutors in the project of sustaining and repairing their disclosing relation, in the face of what cannot be fully known. This need not be a failing of interpersonal life, nor does it mean that disclosure needs to be perfected in some way to reduce the chance of miscommunication or to more fully express oneself. Rather, what cannot be known, what sits outside of that which is disclosed, is important to social experience and interpersonal life. This aspect of disclosure is clear in, for example, Kokanovic's and Philip's cases of disclosure and mental illness, Davis's and Flowers's examination of online disclosures, and Vernon's account of the disclosure strategies of transsexuals. In each of these arenas, disclosure is always framed by that which is not and cannot be told, underlining the interpretive and ethical challenges of what to reveal and what not to, and how to interpret what is revealed and what may not have been.

The authors in this volume also often relied on notions of reciprocity, treating disclosure as a form of exchange that instantiates and stabilises kinds of social ties, resonating with the theoretical and empirical basis of the gift relationship (Mauss 1990 [1950]). When disclosed to, the listener is placed in the social situation of 'response-ability', as the witness of portentous facts. For this reason, something happens to the interaction: relations alter in the face of telling. The teller, through the act of disclosure, makes a statement about his or her relationship to the listener, as much as he or she makes a statement of themselves; the listener is thereby faced with choice, that is, whether or not and how to respond, even if only in some way to acknowledge what has been disclosed. This implies that the response to a disclosure is itself a disclosure of a kind, for it reveals something of the listener such as their attitude towards the discloser or the category of illness or social circumstances that is the subject of the disclosure. Disclosure therefore invites (even provokes) a response. A person who chooses to disclose anticipates the response of the other, and the response shapes the relationship thereafter.

Many of the chapters in this volume, also, made the link between disclosure and personal experience narrative, noting that in both framings of social interaction, telling of oneself implies a subject constructing a story for an audience, both real and imagined. Through this circuit of telling and the transformation of the social relation, disclosure provides a significant means for producing social connectedness.

Disclosure in context

In this volume, we have primarily focused on disclosure as it pertains to intimate life and the social worlds of the discloser and listener, although we have acknowledged that telling of oneself is not restricted to such interactions. The contributing authors to this volume have touched on the practices and ramifications of disclosing to partners, family and others in social worlds and how we negotiate these; but, also, many have reflected on, and addressed, the limited containment of any disclosure. Disclosures travel through personal and other social networks, even when told with a caveat not to tell on.

In this volume, we have also strived to sustain the idea that any analysis of disclosure requires attention to its contexts. Who tells what to whom, and how, is of paramount significance in shaping what disclosure is and can do. Flaherty, Preloran and Browner show that in the context of inherited genetic illness, disclosure operates not as one person conveying information to another, or in relation to a medical practitioner informing his or her patient of a diagnosis, but as a growing awareness among siblings, partners and family groups of a disease that requires explanation. Here, establishing a diagnosis becomes important, not necessarily for what it reveals of the illness or the possible prognosis, but for its ontological value in the social networks of the patient, its implications for those who might have to consider themselves as susceptible, and for the legitimisation of caring relationships. Their work shows that partnership and kinship are important frames that structure how disclosure is enacted and its effects. In a different way, the chapters by Kokanovic and Philip and by Wolf-Meyer, develop disclosure's significance for the workplace. Mental illness and narcolepsy have implications for employment, shaping opportunities and relations with employers and employees, so precipitating the need to disclose at some point, to manage one's illness, and to ensure safety in the workplace; or, alternatively, placing on individuals the difficult burden of not disclosing and preventing exposure.

These examples take this volume's collective analyses close to the orthodox view of disclosure as legally required. But as the authors illustrate in these and other chapters, disclosure is always more than the simple establishment of a fact regarding the person. Root's account of church-based disclosures and non-disclosure of HIV, for example, underlines how a person with HIV infection must navigate myriad social complexities that more or less enable disclosure, even at times foreclosing it. The analysis by Davis and Flowers of online HIV and chlamydia disclosures, too, points out the novel ways in which social contexts can be created to inform intimate others and potential sex partners of one's biomedical status and intentions. Indeed, as they illustrate, in some circumstances it is possible to disclose one's sexual health status without disclosing anything else, or so it seems. And while their example highlights this potential in a mediated world, it is possible in therapeutic settings, for instance, to disclose as an alcoholic, a narcotic user or a gambler in a support group, while other identities – as a parent, partner or worker – are unspoken, rendered irrelevant or private and secret.

One feature of disclosure, as we have elaborated, is that it is not discrete. Disclosures are embedded in social relations. They are contextualised in flows of social interaction. They have settings and choreographies, as in the case of a disclosure from a doctor to a patient of their diagnosis. Disclosures can be taken to infer past and memory, implying also an imagined future, a life of a different valence, post-disclosure. Psychological support often assists those who might need to disclose or others who are thought to benefit from disclosing something difficult, such as mental illness or HIV serostatus (Dyson et al. 2010, Irvine 2011, Kairania et al. 2010, Suthers et al. 2011). The role of the 'helping professionals' in such instances is to script the disclosure. The presumption, here, is that telling is both necessary and good, a vehicle to shift either a psychological state or a social relationship to a new plane. Disclosure is therefore thought to produce closure, at one level and, in so doing, to augur a new beginning.

At the same time, telling of one aspect of one's health may precipitate forms of implied disclosures. HIV, again, is a good example of this. As Root explored in her work, disclosure is carefully considered and at times avoided because of the implied associations it brings of the discloser's sexual behaviour or other aspects of their life they might prefer to keep from others. Disclosure of one aspect of oneself, then, can also stand in for another disclosure. At times too, meaning is given to what is not said, as Squire shows in connection with non-disclosure of HIV serostatus. The non-disclosure of infection can mobilise questions and assumptions of serostatus in social settings where disclosure is expected.

We have made the point in this volume that disclosures are not always singular. They transpire over a life course. While particular disclosures occur at particular moments, they do not exist outside of biographic time. Repeat encounters of the disclosure's interlocutors can embellish, deepen and modify the social effects of a particular disclosure. This process is perhaps most evident in Vernon's account of transsexuals, who reported that managing knowledge of their gender change is repeated at such events as family gatherings or in the workplace. This effect is also discernible in Boddy's research on the family narrative. In this context, prior interviews with the family come to take on different meanings and resonances because of what becomes apparent in a later interview. As life moves, then so do the practice and implications of self-revelation, accentuating the emotional and relational labour that comes with family life, partnering, workplace reputation, and the biographic shaping of the self.

Disclosure as strategy

Another important cross-cutting theme of this collection concerns the strategic way in which disclosers consider what to disclose and why. Kokanovic and Philip show that people with serious mental illness carefully manage what is told to whom, in an effort to reduce prejudice and other negative outcomes. Davis and Flowers show how, in the case of HIV and sexually transmitted infections, disclosure is carefully orchestrated in casual sexual encounters and in the methods of contact tracing operated by sexual health clinics. In these contexts, online and mobile phone technologies provide various and evolving options for visibility and confidentiality.

People make decisions all of the time about what to tell to whom. Boddy's account of family storytelling in Andhra Pradesh reveals how family members collaborated in preserving the viability of the family unit in the face of serious threats. Vernon showed the acute and continuous disclosure dilemmas that face people who have undertaken sex re-assignment. In some instances, disclosure's contingencies seemed overwhelming as one's past in one gender collided with one's chosen gender and its future.

Those who find they wish or need to disclose, or perceive little option but to do so, seek out safe spaces and contexts to tell. This was particularly clear in relation to mental illness, infectious diseases and transsexuality, indicating the symbolic weight of such disclosures. This feature of potentially disruptive disclosures is well known in the literature, which focuses on the benefits and drawbacks of disclosure and how the person who needs to disclose, or has chosen to do so, can be assisted to carry that out without too many negative consequences (see Dyson et al. 2010, Irvine 2011, Kairania et al. 2010, Suthers et al. 2011). Case studies in this volume show that people addressed their self-made disclosures as a feature of social interaction that was more or less volitional, but not, of course, outside the material constraints of their lives. Individuals considered when their diagnoses ought to be disclosed, as was the case for the people with narcolepsy as described by Wolf-Meyer, who had to gauge when it would be prudent to inform employers of the risk they might pose. Individuals also considered what elements of their personal circumstances ought to be conveyed and when. Vernon's account of the complex disclosures of transsexuals demonstrates the articulation of 'on a need to know' rationality, also noted by Squire in connection with HIV disclosures.

These and other less provocative disclosures are marked, at times, by the importance of emotional connection. Seeking disclosure is bound up with a desire to express something of the significance of the relationship between the discloser and the listener(s), in this volume, especially in deeply personal contexts. Disclosure is an exchange of information but it also can have strong affective valence for the interlocutors. These emotional resonances secure and deepen the social connection, adding a layer to the reciprocity and 'response-ability' implied in disclosure, as already discussed. The emotional significance of disclosure and its resonance with the gift relationship is suggestive of its role in late modern societies where social ties are said to be weakened because they exist outside of the traditions and places which previously supported them (Bauman 2003, Beck and Beck-Gernsheim 1995). In this view, disclosure, through its emotional valency and powers of gift, can be take to be more – not less – important to intersubjective experience. Disclosure, through its emotional value in particular, may be one way in which social worlds are made and sustained in the face of the loss of those structures which bound us together in the past.

Deciding not to disclose is always immanent in the practice of telling. Non-disclosures can be produced from the disclosures of others. Root's examination of HIV disclosure practices in African communities demonstrates how some decide to not speak of their HIV serostatus after observing the aftermath of someone else's disclosure. Disclosure practices are shaped, then, by some sense of there being more than one interlocutor, that to disclose is to alter one's social presence in a collective context and even that one's disclosure could become a public matter. The vicarious learning enabled by the disclosures of others indicates one way in which telling and revelation inform public life, a point we take up below.

Disclosure and biography

Disclosure has a significant relationship with biography. A health event such as diagnosis of a disease or infection, or the advent of surgery, is a moment in the life course that can transform one's identity and social worlds. Telling of these events is one way in which subjects can come to know of themselves and confer meaning on experience, furthering the construction of a life story. Boddy's analysis of her family's story shows how the partial and titrated disclosure of major events – the death of one son and the violence of the father – are vital for understanding what is happening for this family. The partial and nuanced disclosures of the mother and child establish the family's past and present and their collective identity as resilient and determined, but not without signalling also the effects in the life of the child interviewed, forced as he is to set aside play and take on a role in the family's day-to-day survival. The participants in the research of Flaherty, Preloran and Browner tell of seeking out diagnosis for what it may offer by way of explanation for distressing symptoms; the diagnosis, and its recounting to others, confirms and validates rather than depletes or despoils. Disclosure operates here to lay claim to biography, imposing order where that may be threatened.

Disclosure is also deeply temporalising. It marks before and after. As many of the authors in this volume have noted, disclosures cannot be retracted; disclosers are acutely aware of this when they disclose or when they reflect on what might happen if they do so. Disclosures, then, transform existence, in the sense that they mark a biographical moment in the life of the discloser but also because they create a 'watershed' in the social relation of discloser and listener(s). This aspect of disclosure resonates strongly with the idea that disclosure is 'onto-performative'. Biographies are made in their telling and disclosure of one's health status is here a key element.

As with biography, disclosures have their moment in history. Some disclosures become redundant or negated because of shifts in the life course and in culture, making them unnecessary or unintelligible. Ken Plummer (1995) has explored coming out in this way, showing that disclosure of homosexual orientation became possible once individuals felt that they would be able to make such disclosures. In more recent times, however, the coming-out story seems less relevant (Altman 2013). This implies that there are points in history when telling is enabled interpersonally and culturally, but that also some aspects of self cease to possess the necessity of disclosure and lack the cultural weight they previously possessed. Here, we are suggesting not only that some things lose cultural salience, and no longer need to be told, but, also, that the status attached to such disclosures, marking an individual as distinctive in a particular way, is lost.

Disclosure and civic life

The argument we have developed in this volume implies that disclosure has implications for citizenship and public life. As noted, some forms of disclosure are legal requirements, for example, in a workplace where one's illness may pose a risk to co-workers or clients, or in public health where it is illegal in some jurisdictions to fail to disclose an infectious disease such as HIV to a sexual partner. The private world of the discloser, and the social relations they seek to construct with those who might care to listen to their story, can also be tied into citizenly rights and responsibilities. To disclose of oneself, however, is to destroy that which was hitherto secret, to make the private slightly less so. Modern societies, too, are deeply invested in what private matters are also of public interest and disclosures in social life sit against the backdrop of media-scapes where so much of what is private is public fare.

Celebrity disclosures are perhaps iconic of the contemporary interest in private lives. Catherine Zeta-Jones's bipolar disorder (Kirkova 2013), Angelina Jolie's prophylactic mastectomy (Payne 2013) and Stephen Fry's breakdown (Rayner 2013), like multiple public stories of uncontrolled alcohol and drug abuse, sexual abuse and violence, are well-publicised if short-lived health events. These media stories are not unlike the disclosures we have discussed in this volume, though they have a highly editorialised, parodic quality that opens up questions of the extent to which they are truly revealing of the lives of the celebrities. The spectacular visibility of these disclosures could be taken to be a kind of mask for the real, a way of hiding or deflecting attention and therefore securing privacy and preserving secrets. Such stories often also redeem the discloser, providing the means for bio-graphical restitution or some other kind of repair of the moral self (Frank 1995). Stories like these, too, are strongly inflected with pedagogical value, serving as lessons for all of us on the virtues and pitfalls of disclosure and the need to disclose along the road to recovery. Improved mental health and psychological wellbeing are routinely represented as the outcomes of dis-closure, and alternative accounts of disclosure as foolhardy or unnecessary are rare. Such mediated stories indicate that public disclosure is a mode of spectatorship where the biographic events of celebrities are offered so that they can be lived vicariously. Identifying with these disclosures – 'there but for the grace of God go I' – implies that they function as parables, providing readers and viewers with a moral education for how one can and should cope with serious health conditions. Celebrity disclosures thus provide an emotional and ethical template for domestic disclosures.

As Ken Plummer (2003) has shown, however, the making of the private public is not restricted to celebrities as the private lives of everyday citizens are increasingly open to public scrutiny. Reality television programmes play with this breakdown of public and private, celebrity and domestic. The Australian television programme *RPA* (Channel Nine, Australia) features lengthy quasi-documentary stories of individuals facing medical interventions and surgery at Sydney's Royal Prince Alfred Hospital. We can therefore be said to live in a celebrity- and citizen-disclosing culture where self-revelation and the circulation of private lives in public life is constantly replayed. This idea that the personal is of public interest imbues all disclosure practices with the resonances of spectatorship and consumption. Everyone has before them the chance to be on show, to be a narcissist, even if they do not get the chance to have their story displayed in a magazine or on television. Perhaps it is even a requirement of modern life to narcissistically make oneself available to others.

In the era of Facebook and Wikileaks, too, personal and anonymous disclosures take place and overlap, furthering the ontological troubles for any definite notion of public versus private. As Davis and Flowers have illustrated in connection with media technologies, some disclosures are made in relatively public ways, with a community of intelligibility, rather than a single listener, in mind. Flaherty, Preloran and Browner make the point too that the disclosure of diagnosis of Huntington's disease involves family groups, showing that the model of disclosure as a private matter for the individual is untenable or, at least, that the idea of private is malleable.

As noted, there are also civic requirements that one disclose. People with sleep disorders find that they are compelled to disclose when it may cost them their jobs. People with mental illness disclose in the workplace to lay claim to sickness benefits but at the risk of their careers. Transsexuals find that establishing their gender can lead to crises of identity in the workplace or in marriage. People with HIV also find that they are expected and in some instances required to disclose in ways that may compromise their social standing. As contributors to this volume have shown, the civic and public dimensions of disclosure depend on the nature of the disease or condition, social expectations, responsibility and risk to others. Underlying these questions of citizenship that pertain to disclosure, there is a concern with whether or not the person reveals the truth about themselves. This begs the question of the nature of truth, of course, and the possibility of a single truth about the self that might, or should, be shared.

Disclosure and knowledge

Disclosure, then, is implied in the production of knowledge regarding subjective life and research ethics. The later chapters in this volume in particular have taken up questions of the knowledge politics and regimes of truth that are implied in practices of disclosure. Wolf-Meyer examines disclosure in relation to ethnographic inquiry, exploring the dilemmas faced by a researcher when reporting on their observations and other data and adhering to the requirements of research ethics committees to do no harm to research participants and to protect their identities. In the same way as disclosure is enacted in social life, the disclosures made in a research setting, including by the research participant explicitly to the researcher, and the disclosures that the researcher ought to make in relation to their conduct of the research enterprise, are deeply contextual and strategic. Wolf-Meyer also takes the step of connecting this critique with a more general one of verisimilitude and the ethnographic representation of lives. Playing with varying degrees of anonymisation and interpretive representation of the human condition, Wolf-Meyer points to enduring questions regarding research ethics and epistemology. Disclosure is a flashpoint for knowledge production of the human condition, densely imbued with questions of ethical conduct, truth and representation.

Vernon's chapter takes up questions of truth and representation in connection with gender. Questioning the taken for granted status of natal gender, Vernon raises questions too of what counts as truth in a disclosure of one's gender re-assignment surgery. A dominant cissexual norm, as she describes this, is that true gender is set at birth, an assumption that under-mines transsexual claims that their chosen gender is their true gender.

Vernon's analysis demonstrates that a transsexual woman's claim to truth troubles prevailing assumptions of what is true about one's body and mind. Disclosure, at least in this case, is therefore already bound up with standpoint epistemology. From the point of view of some transsexual women, telling the truth founders on the cissexual position that natality, or the pre-sex reassignment surgery body, should rule gender truth, though Vernon also demonstrates that a mix of biological determinism and socialisation theory informs the cissexual point of view. Disclosure, then, reveals the political dynamics of truth, or more properly the agonistic relations of different and contradictory regimes of knowledge production regarding truth, of gender and other matters of experience.

Squire extends this critique of telling and its relation to knowledge through a discussion of HIV disclosure's mercurial qualities. Telling someone of one's HIV serostatus is never just the transmission of knowledge regarding the outcome of the HIV antibody test. To say one is HIV positive or HIV negative implies too much knowledge, for it suggests practices and histories thought to be related to the need to test for HIV, in general, and an HIV positive test outcome, in particular. It invites speculation; the listener is open to further disclosure or, equally as telling, withdraws and resists further knowledge. Importantly, though, HIV disclosure also hardly reveals anything that matters, since people are always more than their diagnosis. Health and illness disclosures in general share in this problematic of knowledge of the subject. Any biomedical truth is liable to mobilise inferences and occlusions that give intersubjective life its particular form. This is perhaps medicalisation at its most profound; speaking of one's health and illness expands the resonant and associational effects of biomedical forms of knowledge in social existence. As contributors to this volume have indicated, how to disclose so that it does not matter or matters less was an aspiration shared by many of those affected by health concerns, but finding a way to achieve this – to tell without being subsumed by it – evaded them nonetheless. Reflecting on them and dissecting their effects was one way of addressing the cultural circumstances of disclosure, and perhaps this was one means by which individuals were able to work towards that point when a particular fact (a medical diagnosis, a biographic point) might become less troublesome, even redundant. Disclosure, however, is itself a form of knowledge that is self-perpetuating. For instance, disclosing in ways that have no impacts in one's social world is liable to go unnoticed, that is, it is not a 'disclosure' at all.

With the other chapters in this volume, Wolf-Meyer, Vernon and Squire point towards a 'disclosure-sensitive' literacy for social inquiry. Revealing oneself – in a research project or in social life – is not equivalent to knowledge shared. How one responds to disclosed knowledge raises questions of representation and ethics, salient across research and social life. Truth claims are political, lending disclosure political value that goes beyond the strategic interpersonal dimensions already noted. Disclosure is never all that needs to be known, as it can say too much or far too little. These qualities of disclosure are important to recognise in research that seeks to investigate it, in efforts to assist people to make effective disclosures and protect them from negative effects, and in research inquiry in general.

* * *

We have offered a view on disclosure in health and illness that resists reducing it to a simple utterance of a biomedical label in the clinical encounter or in other social contexts. Disclosures can be like this, of course, but the transmission of self-knowledge is always more.

The case studies of this volume have come from the global North and South, and have addressed poverty and family violence, HIV and sexually transmitted infections, inherited neurological disease, narcolepsy and transsexualism; through their diversity, they demonstrate disclosure's substantive complexities. By tying disclosure to social theories of identity and relationality, we have established the importance of context and strategy for how we understand it. We have also elaborated on disclosure's resonances with biography and in civic life. And we have pointed to the politics of truth and representation that are also implied in the investigation of disclosure. As noted, we have drawn on these empirical and conceptual resources in an effort to pursue a 'disclosure-sensitive' literacy for social inquiry. Several of our authors have written of how disclosure might be emptied of its negative consequences, or of how it might be exhausted of its troublesome effects for disclosers and listeners. And this is certainly the aspiration of research and social support that aims to assist people to make disclosures in ways that help them. Contemporary mores, however, give the impression that knowledge of the self is an important aspect of the knowledge economy, with personal information attracting value and able to be sold on to interested parties. Public administration expects that citizens be willing to disclose personal information to inform how we are to be governed, not least in the area of health and illness. Neoliberal public health and preventive medicine programmes, too, assume both that individuals know themselves and that they make known their selves to others to intervene effectively. Disclosure is a seemingly ubiquitous imperative, yet its implications, as chapters in this volume demonstrate, are profound. The critical perspectives on disclosure we have offered, therefore, are important tools for social inquiry into contemporary turnings in health and illness, and beyond.

References

Chapter 1: Telling points

Ashforth, A. and N. Nattrass. 2005. Ambiguities of 'culture' and the antiretroviral rollout in South Africa. *Social Dynamics: A Journal of the Centre for African Studies* 31, 2: 285–303.

Astbury-Ward, E., O. Parry and R. Carnwell. 2012. Stigma, abortion, and disclosure: Findings from a qualitative study. *Journal of Sexual Medicine* 9, 12: 3137–3147.

Australian Federation of AIDS Organizations. 2013. http://www.afao.org.au/about-hiv/hiv-and-the-law/disclosure/gay-men-and-hiv-disclosure.

Bennett, E. S. 1999. Soft truth: Ethics and cancer in Northeast Thailand. *Anthropology & Medicine* 14, 1: 15–26.

Bharadwaj, A. 2003. Why adoption is not an option in India: The visibility of infertility, the secrecy of donor insemination, and other cultural complexities. *Social Science & Medicine* 56, 9: 1867–80.

Chhim, S. 2012. Baksbat (broken courage): A trauma-based cultural syndrome in Cambodia. *Medical Anthropology* 32, 2: 160–73.

Crook, T. 1999. Growing knowledge in Bolivip, Papua New Guinea. *Oceania* 69, 4: 225–42.

Daftary, A. 2012. HIV and tuberculosis: The construction and management of double stigma. *Social Science & Medicine* 74, 10: 1512–9.

De Zorda, S. 2012. In search of pleasure and respect: Biomedical contraceptive technologies in Bahia Brazil. In L. Manderson (ed.) *Technologies of Sexuality, Identity and Sexual Health*, pp. 16–34. London: Routledge.

Den Heijer, M. 2013. Diplomatic asylum and the Assange case. *Leiden Journal of International Law* 26, 2: 399–425.

Foucault, M. 1978. *The History of Sexuality*, Volume 1. New York: Random House.

Funabashi, Y. and K. Kitazawa 2012. Fukushima in review: A complex disaster, a disastrous response. *Bulletin of the Atomic Scientists* 68, 2: 9–21.

George, K. M. 1993. Dark trembling: Ethnographic notes on secrecy and concealment in highland Sulawesi. *Anthropological Quarterly* 66, 4: 230–9.

Goffman, E. 1959. *The Presentation of Self in Everyday Life*. New York: Doubleday.

—— 1963. *Stigma: Notes on the Management of Spoiled Identity*. Englewood Cliffs NJ: Prentice Hall.

Hanssen, I. 2004. From human ability to ethical principle: An intercultural perspective on autonomy. *Medicine, Health Care, and Philosophy* 7, 3: 269–79.

Hardon, A. and D. Posel. 2012. Secrecy as embodied practice: Beyond the confessional imperative introduction. *Culture, Health and Sexuality* 14, SI: S1–S13.

Harris, L. H., M. Debbink, L. Martin et al. 2011. Dynamics of stigma in abortion work: Findings from a pilot study of the Providers Share Workshop. *Social Science & Medicine* 73, 7: 1062–70.

Hertogh, C. M., B. A. The, B. M. Miesen and J. A. Eefsting. 2004. Truth telling and truthfulness in the care for patients with advanced dementia: An ethnographic study in Dutch nursing homes. *Social Science & Medicine* 59, 8: 1685–93.

Holden, K. 2012. http://www.baliadvertiser.biz/articles/ubudwriters/2012/kate_holden.html.

Hollingsworth, L. D., D. Swick and Y. J. Choi. 2013. The role of positive and negative social interactions in child custody outcomes: Voices of US women with serious mental illness. *Qualitative Social Work* 12, 2: 153–69.

Hymer, S. 1995. Therapeutic and redemptive aspects of religious confession. *Journal of Religion & Health* 34, 1: 41–54.

Kaufert, J. M. 1999. Cultural mediation in cancer diagnosis and end of life decision making: The experience of Aboriginal patients in Canada. *Anthropology & Medicine* 6, 3: 405–21.

Kidwell, M. and E. G. Martinez. 2010. 'Let me tell you about myself': A method for suppressing subject talk in a 'soft accusation' interrogation. *Discourse Studies* 12, 1: 65–89.

Kokanovic, R. and L. Manderson. 2006. Social support and self-management of type 2 diabetes among immigrant Australian women. *Chronic Illness* 2, 4: 291–301.

Leveson, B. 2012. *The Report into the Culture, Practices and Ethics of the Press.* London: The Stationery Office.

Martel, J. 2010. Remorse and the production of truth. *Punishment & Society: International Journal of Penology* 12, 4: 414–37.

Munro, I. and J. Randall. 2007. 'I don't know what I'm doing, how about you?': Discourse and identity in practitioners dealing with the survivors of childhood sexual abuse. *Organization* 14, 6: 887–907.

Murray, E. J., V. A. Bond, B. J. Marais et al. 2013. High levels of vulnerability and anticipated stigma reduce the impetus for tuberculosis diagnosis in Cape Town, South Africa. *Health Policy and Planning* 28, 4: 410–18.

Niehaus, I. 2014. Treatment literacy, therapeutic efficacy, and antiretroviral drugs: Notes from Bushbuckridge, South Africa. *Medical Anthropology*. In press.

Okri, B. 1991. *The Famished Road.* London: Jonathan Cape.

Padilla, M., D. Castellanos, V. Guilamo-Ramos, A. M. Reyes, L. E. Sanchez Marte and M. Arredondo Soriano. 2008. Stigma, social inequality, and HIV risk disclosure among Dominican male sex workers. *Social Science & Medicine* 67, 3: 380–8.

Parle, J. and F. Scorgie. 2012. Bewitching Zulu women: Umhayizo, gender, and witchcraft in KwaZulu-Natal. *South African Historical Journal* 64, 4: 852–75.

Petryna, A. 2003. *Life Exposed: Biological Citizens after Chernobyl.* Princeton NJ: Princeton University Press.

Readings, J., L. Blake, P. Casey et al. 2011. Secrecy, disclosure and everything in-between: Decisions of parents of children conceived by donor insemination, egg donation and surrogacy. *Reproductive Biomedicine Online* 22, 5: 485–95

Root, R. 2010. Situating experiences of HIV-related stigma in Swaziland. *Global Public Health* 5, 5: 523–38.

Rose, D., K. Trevillion, A. Woodall, C. Morgan, G. Feder and L. Howard. 2011. Barriers and facilitators of disclosures of domestic violence by mental health service users: Qualitative study. *British Journal of Psychiatry* 198, 3: 189–94.

Sargent, C. and L. Kitobi. 2012. Contraceptive secrets: Body battles among North and West African migrants in Paris. In L. Manderson (ed.) *Technologies of Sexuality, Identity and Sexual Health*, pp. 35–54. London: Routledge.

Scorgie, F., D. Nakato, E. Harper et al. 2013. 'We are despised in the hospitals': Sex workers' experiences of accessing health care in four African countries. *Culture, Health and Sexuality* 15, 4: 450–65.

Seeman, M.V. 2013. When and how should I tell? Personal disclosure of a schizophrenia diagnosis in the context of intimate relationships. *Psychiatric Quarterly* 84, 1: 93–102.

Shellenberg, K. M., A. M. Moore, A. Bankole et al. 2011. Social stigma and disclosure about induced abortion: Results from an exploratory study. *Global Public Health* 6, SI: S111–S125.

Tenkorang, E. Y., S. O. Gyimah, E. Maticka-Tyndale et al. 2011. Superstition, witchcraft and HIV prevention in sub-Saharan Africa: The case of Ghana. *Culture, Health & Sexuality* 13, 9: 1001–14.

Tonda, J. 2001. From the human body to the body politic: Scope of divine healing in Congo. *Social Compass* 48, 3: 403–20.

van Berkell, D., A. Candido and W. H. Pijffers. 2007. Becoming a mother by nonanonymous egg donation: Secrecy and the relationship between egg recipient, egg donor and egg donation child. *Journal of Psychosomatic Obstetrics and Gynecology* 28, 2: 97–104.

van der Sijpt, E. 2012. 'The vagina does not talk': Conception concealed or deliberately disclosed in eastern Cameroon. *Culture, Health & Sexuality* 14, S1: S81–S94.

Westad, C. and D. McConnell. 2012. Child welfare involvement of mothers with mental health issues. *Community Mental Health Journal* 48, 1: 29–37.

Wilhelm-Solomon, M. 2013. The Priest's Soldiers: HIV therapies, health identities, and forced encampment in Northern Uganda. *Medical Anthropology* 32, 3: 227–46.

Wyndham, M. and P. Read. 2010. From state terrorism to state errorism: Post-Pinochet Chile's long search for truth and justice. *Public Historian* 32, 1: 31–44.

Youatt, E., M. Debbink, L. Martin et al. 2012. 'Can't talk about work, can't talk about my relationship': Sexual minority abortion providers cope with stigma and identity disclosure. *Contraception* 86, 3: 304.

Chapter 2: Stories told in passing?

Balagopalan, S. 2011. Introduction: Children's lives and the Indian context. *Childhood* 18, 3: 291–7.

Bauman, R. 1986. *Story, Performance and Event. Contextual Studies of Oral Narrative*. Cambridge UK: Cambridge University Press.

Boddy, J. and M. Smith. 2008. Asking the experts: Developing and validating parental diaries to assess children's minor injuries. *International Journal of Social Research Methodology* 11, 1: 63–77.

Bruner, J. 1990. *Acts of Meaning*. Cambridge MA: Harvard University Press.

—— 1991. The narrative construction of reality. *Critical Inquiry* 18: 1–21.

Buitelaar, M. 2006. 'I am the ultimate challenge': Accounts of intersectionality in the life-story of a well-known daughter of Moroccan migrant workers in the Netherlands. *European Journal of Women's Studies* 13, 3: 259–76.

Crivello, G., V. Morrow and N. Streuli. 2013. *Young Lives Qualitative Fieldwork Guide. Round Three (2010/2011). Technical Note 29.* Oxford UK: Young Lives.

Crivello, G., V. Morrow and E. Wilson. 2013. *Young Lives Longitudinal Qualitative Research. A Guide for Researchers. Technical Note 26.* Oxford UK: Young Lives.

Economic and Social Research Council. 2010. *Framework for Research Ethics.* Swindon UK: ESRC.

Fox, C. 2008. Postcolonial dilemmas in narrative research. *Compare: A Journal of Comparative and International Education* 38, 3: 335–47.

Galab, S., P. P. Reddy and R. Himaz. 2008. *Young Lives Round 2 Survey Report Initial Findings: Andhra Pradesh, India.* Oxford UK: Young Lives.

Gillis, J. R. 1996. *A World of Their Own Making: Myth, Ritual, and the Quest for Family Values.* New York: Basic Books.

Halkier, B., T. Katz-Gerro and L. Martens. 2011. Applying practice theory to the study of consumption: Theoretical and methodological considerations. *Journal of Consumer Culture* 11, 1: 3–13.

Hargreaves, T. 2011. Practice-ing behaviour change: Applying social practice theory to pro-environmental behaviour change. *Journal of Consumer Culture* 11, 1: 79–99.

Hermans, H. J. M. 2003. The construction and reconstruction of a dialogical self. *Journal of Constructivist Psychology* 16, 2: 89–130.

Hitchings, R. 2011. People can talk about their practices. *Area* 44, 1: 61–7.

Hulme, M. 2009. *Why We Disagree About Climate Change: Understanding Controversy, Inaction and Opportunity.* Cambridge UK: Cambridge University Press.

Langellier, K. M. 1999. Personal narrative, performance, performativity: Two or three things I know for sure. *Text and Performance Quarterly* 19, 2: 125–44.

McAdam, D. P. 1993. *The Stories We Live By: Personal Myths and the Making of the Self.* New York: Guilford Press.

Moran, J. 2005. *Reading the Everyday.* London: Routledge.

Morgan, D. 2011. Locating 'family practices'. *Sociological Research Online* 16, 4: 14.

Morrow, V. and U. Vennam. 2009. Children Combining Work and Education in Cottonseed Production in Andhra Pradesh: Implications for Discourses of Children's Rights in India. *Young Lives Working Paper 50.* Oxford UK: Young Lives.

Miller, D. 2012. *Consumption and Its Consequences.* Cambridge UK: Polity.

Myers, N. and J. Kent. 2003. New consumers: The influence of affluence on the environment. *Proceedings of the National Academy of Sciences* 100, 8: 4963–8.

OED Online. 2013. 'disclosure, n.' Oxford: Oxford University Press. http://www.oed.com/view/Entry/53779?redirectedFrom=disclosure.

Phoenix, A. 2008. Analysing narrative contexts. In M. Andrews, C. Squire and M. Tamboukou (eds) *Doing Narrative Research*, pp. 64–77. London: Sage.

Pink, S. 2009. *Doing Sensory Ethnography.* London: Sage.

Ramsay, T. and L. Manderson. 2011. Resilience, spirituality, and post-traumatic growth: Reshaping the effects of climate change. In I. Weissbecker (ed.) *Climate Change and Human Well-being: Global Challenges and Opportunities*, pp. 165–84. London: Springer.

Reckwitz, A. 2002. Toward a theory of social practices. A development in culturalist theorizing. *European Journal of Social Theory* 5, 2: 243–63.

Revi, A. 2008. Climate change risk: An adaptation and mitigation agenda for Indian cities. *Environment and Urbanisation* 20, 1: 207–29.

Riessman, C. K. 2000. Stigma and everyday resistance practices: Childless women in South India. *Gender and Society* 14: 111–35.

—— 2003. Analysis of personal narratives. In J. A. Holstein and J. F. Gubrium (eds) *Inside Interviewing: New Lenses, New Concerns*. London: Sage.

Schatzki, T. R. 2001. Introduction. Practice theory. In T. R. Schatzki, K. K. Cetina and E. von Savigny (eds) *The Practice Turn in Contemporary Theory*, pp. 1–14. Oxford UK: Routledge.

Scott, S. 2009. *Making Sense of Everyday Life*. Cambridge UK: Polity Press.

Shove, E. 2010. Social theory and climate change. Questions often, sometimes and not yet asked. *Theory, Culture & Society* 27, 2–3: 277–88.

Squire, C. 2005. Reading narratives. *Group Analysis* 38, 1: 91–107.

—— 2008. Experience-centred and culturally-oriented approaches to narrative. In M. Andrews, C. Squire and M. Tamboukou (eds) *Doing Narrative Research*, pp. 42–63. London: Sage.

Vennam, U. and A. Komanduri. 2009. *Young Lives Qualitative Research: Round 1 – India*. Oxford UK: Young Lives.

Warde, A. 2005. Consumption and theories of practice. *Journal of Consumer Culture* 5, 2: 131–53.

WHO. 2013. *Global and Regional Estimates of Violence Against Women: Prevalence and Health Effects of Intimate Partner Violence and Non-partner Sexual Violence*. Geneva: World Health Organization.

Chapter 3: Being HIV positive

Adam, B. 2011. Epistemic fault lines in biomedical and social approaches to HIV prevention. *Journal of the International AIDS Society* 14, suppl. 2: S1–9.

African Religious Health Assets Programme. 2006. *Appreciating Assets: The Contribution of Religion to Universal Access in Africa. Report for the World Health Organization*. Cape Town, South Africa: African Religious Health Assets Programme.

Bastos, C. 1999. *Global Responses to AIDS: Science in Emergency*. Bloomington IN: Indiana University Press.

Becker, G. 2004. Phenomenology of health and illness. In C. Ember and M. Ember (eds) *The World's Cultures, Encyclopedia of Medical Anthropology*, pp. 125–36. New York: Kluwer Academic/Plenum Publishers.

Booth, A. 1983. *Swaziland: Tradition and Change in a Southern African Kingdom*. Boulder CO: Westview Press.

Buseh, A., L. Glass and B. McElmurry. 2002. Cultural and gender issues related to HIV/AIDS prevention in rural Swaziland: A focus group analysis. *Health Care for Women International* 23, 2: 173–84.

Campbell, C. and H. Deacon. 2006. Introduction: Unravelling the contexts of stigma: from internalisation to resistance to change. *Journal of Community & Applied Social Psychology* 16, 6: 411–17.

Centres for Disease Control. 2012. *Swaziland Factsheet*. http://www.cdc.gov/globalhealth/countries/swaziland/pdf/swaziland.pdf.

Chandra, P., S. Deepthivarma and V. Manjula. 2003. Disclosure of HIV infection in South India: Patterns, reasons and reactions. *AIDS Care* 15, 2: 207–15.

Chaudoir, S. and J. Fisher. 2010. The disclosure processes model: Understanding disclosure decision-making and post-disclosure outcomes among people living with a concealable stigmatised identity. *Psychological Bulletin* 136, 2: 236–56.

Chaudoir, S., J. Fisher and J. Simoni. 2011. Understanding HIV disclosure: A review and application of the Disclosure Processes Model. *Social Science & Medicine* 72, 10: 1618–29.

Colvin, C. 2011. HIV/AIDS, chronic diseases and globalisation. *Globalization and Health* 7: 31. http://www.ncbi.nlm.nih.gov/pmc/articles/PMC3179713/.

Commonwealth Local Government Forum. [No date] *The local government system in Swaziland.* http://www.clgf.org.uk/userfiles/1/files/Swaziland%20local%20 government%20profile%202011-12.pdf.

Csordas, T. 1990. Embodiment as a paradigm for anthropology. *Ethos* 18, 1: 5–47.

Deacon, H. 2006. Towards a sustainable theory of health-related stigma: Lessons from the HIV/AIDS literature. *Journal of Community & Applied Social Psychology* 16: 418–25.

Dlamini, P., D. Wantland, L. Makoae, M. Chirwa, T. Kohi, M. Greef et al. 2009. HIV stigma and missed medications in HIV-positive people in five African countries. *AIDS Patient Care and STDS* 23, 5: 377–87.

Earnshaw, V. and S. Chaudoir. 2009. From conceptualizing to measuring HIV stigma: A review of HIV stigma mechanism measure. *AIDS Behavior* 13, 6: 1160–77.

Farmer, P. 1999. *Infection and Inequalities: The Modern Plagues.* Berkeley CA: University of California Press.

Government of Swaziland. [No date] *The Constitution of the Kingdom of Swaziland.* http://www.gov.sz/images/stories/Constitution%20of%20%20SD-2005A001.pdf.

Greef, M., R. Phetlhu, L. Makoae, P. Dlamini, W. Holzemer, J. Naidoo, T. Kohi, L. Uys and M. Chirwa. 2008. Disclosure of HIV status: Experiences and perceptions of persons living with HIV/AIDS and nurses involved in their care in Africa. *Qualitative Health Research* 18, 3: 311–24.

Green, E., C. Dlamini, N. C. D'Errico, A. Ruark and Z. Duby. 2009. Mobilising indigenous resources for anthropologically designed HIV-prevention and behaviour-change interventions in southern Africa. *African Journal of AIDS Research* 8, 4: 389–400.

Hickel, J. 2012. Neoliberal plague: The political economy of HIV transmission in Swaziland. *Journal of Southern African Studies* 38, 3: 513–29.

Holzemer, W., L. Uys, L. Makoae, A. Stewart, R. Phetlhu, P. Dlamini, M. Greef, T. Kohi, M. Chirwa, Y. Cuca and J. Naidoo. 2007. A conceptual model for HIV/AIDS stigma from five African countries. *Journal of Advanced Nursing* 58, 6: 541–51.

Integrated Regional Information Networks (IRIN). 2009. *Swaziland: A culture that encourages HIV/AIDS.* 15 April. http://www.refworld.org/docid/49e6ef2dc.html.

——— 2012. *Swaziland: HIV stigma still a barrier.* http://www.irinnews.org/report/ 96761/swaziland-hiv-stigma-still-a-barrier.

International Fund for Agricultural Development. 2013. *Rural Poverty Portal. Rural Poverty in the Kingdom of Swaziland.* http://www.ruralpovertyportal.org/ country/home/tags/swaziland#.

Irving, A. 2011. Strange distance: Towards an anthropology of interior dialogue. *Medical Anthropology Quarterly* 25, 1: 22–44.

Joint United Nations Programme on HIV/AIDS. 2012. *Swaziland: HIV stigma still a barrier.* http://www.irinnews.org/report/96761/swaziland-hiv-stigma-still-a-barrier.

Kaufman. S. 1988. Toward a phenomenology of boundaries in medicine: Chronic illness experience in the case of stroke. *Medical Anthropology Quarterly* 2, 4: 338–54.

Kiene, S., M. Bateganya, R. Wanyenze, H. Lule, H. Nantabe and M. Stein. 2010. Initial outcomes of provider-initiated routine HIV testing and counseling during outpatient care at a rural Ugandan hospital: Risky sexual behavior, partner HIV testing, disclosure, and HIV care seeking. *AIDS Patient Care and STDS* 24, 2: 117–26.

Kingdom of Swaziland. 2012. *Swaziland Country Report on Monitoring the Political Declaration on HIV/AIDS.* UNAIDS. https://www.unaids.org/en/data analysis/knowyourresponse/countryprogressreports/2012countries/ce_SZ_ Narrative_Report[1].pdf.

Klaits, F. 2010. *Death in a Church of Life: Moral Passion during Botswana's Time of AIDS.* Berkeley CA: University of California Press.

Kippax, S. 2012. Effective HIV prevention: The indispensable role of social science. *Journal of the International AIDS Society* 15, 17357: 1–8.

Kleinman, A. 1988. *The Illness Narratives: Suffering, Healing, and the Human Condition.* New York: Basic Books.

Knibbe, K. and P. Versteeg. 2008. Assessing phenomenology in anthropology: Lessons from the study of religion and experience. *Critique of Anthropology* 28, 1: 47–62.

Kuper, A. 1980. Symbolic dimensions of the Southern Bantu homestead. *Africa: Journal of the International African Institute* 50, 1: 8–23.

Kuper, H. 1986 [1963]. *The Swazi: A South African Kingdom.* New York: Holt, Rinehart, and Winston.

Leclerc-Madlala, S. 2008. Age-disparate and intergenerational sex in southern Africa: The dynamics of hyper-vulnerability. *AIDS* 22, suppl. 4: S17–S25.

Leliveld, A. 1994. The impact of labour migration on the Swazi rural homestead as solidarity group. *Focaal* 22/23: 177–97.

Link, B. and J. Phelan. 2001. Conceptualizing stigma. *Annual Review of Sociology* 27, 1: 363–85.

Lopez, K. and D. Willis. 2004. Descriptive versus interpretive phenomenology: Their contributions to nursing knowledge. *Qualitative Health Research* 14, 5: 726–35.

Lucas, N. 2005. The women's movement in Swaziland: Look how far we've come! *OPENSPACE* 1, 1: 62–3 (a publication of the Open Society Initiative of Southern Africa [OSISA], Johannesburg, South Africa). http://www.osisa.org/publications/ OPENSPACE_1_1.

MacQueen, K. 2011. Commentary. Framing the social in biomedical HIV prevention trials: a 20-year retrospective. *Journal of the International AIDS Society* 14, Suppl. 2: S3.

Manyatsi, A. 2005. Small-scale Irrigated Agriculture and Food Scurity in Swaziland. Paper presented at WARFSA/Waternet Symposium, Ezulwini, Swaziland. http:// www.bscw.ihe.nl/pub/bscw.cgi/d2606552/Manyatsi-Warfsa.pdf.

Marshall, P. 1992. Anthropology and bioethics. *Medical Anthropology Quarterly* 6, 1: 49–73.

Medley, A., C. Garcia-Moreno, S. McGill and S. Maman. 2004. Rates, barriers and outcomes of HIV serostatus disclosure among women in developing countries: Implications for prevention of mother-to-child transmission programmes. *Bulletin of the World Health Organization* 82: 299–307.

Miller, A. and D. Rubin. 2007. Motivations and methods for self-disclosure of HIV seropositivity in Nairobi, Kenya. *AIDS Behavior* 11, 5: 687–97.

Miller, J. 1982. *History and Human Existence from Marx to Merleau-Ponty*. Berkeley CA: University of California Press. UC Press E-Books Collection, 1982–2004. http://publishing.cdlib.org/ucpressebooks/view?docId=ft2489n82k&chunk.id=d0e5027&toc.id=d0e4866&brand=ucpress.

Ministry of Health and Social Welfare (Swaziland). 2008. *Draft National Strategy for HIV/AIDS-Related Stigma and Discrimination*. Mbabane Swaziland: Ministry of Health and Social Welfare.

Moses S. and M. Tomlinson. 2012. The fluidity of disclosure: A longitudinal exploration of women's experience and understanding of HIV disclosure in the context of pregnancy and early motherhood. *AIDS Care*. Epub ahead of print. PubMed PMID: 23110311.

Ngubane, H. 1983. The Swazi homestead. In F. D. Vletter (ed.) *The Swazi Rural Homestead*, ch. 3. Kwaluseni Swaziland: University of Swaziland Social Science Research Unit.

Nolen, S. 2007. Where have all the Swazis gone? *The Globe and Mail*, 22 December: A18.

Norman, A., M. Chopra and S. Kadiyala. 2007. Factors related to HIV disclosure in 2 South African communities. *American Journal of Public Health* 97, 10: 1775–81.

Ntsimane, R. 2006. To disclose or not to disclose: An appraisal of the memory box project as a safe space for disclosure of HIV-positive status. *Journal of Theology for Southern Africa* 125: 7–20.

Obermeyer, C., P. Baijal and E. Pegurri. 2011. Facilitating HIV disclosure across diverse settings: A review. *American Journal of Public Health* 101, 6: 1011–23.

Obeyesekere, G. 1985. Depression, Buddhism, and the work of culture in Sri Lanka. In A. Kleinman and B. Good (eds) *Culture and Depression*, pp. 134–52. Berkeley: University of California Press.

Ogden, J. and L. Nyblade. 2005. Common at its core: HIV-related stigma across contexts. *International Center for Research on Women*. http://www.icrw.org/files/publications/Common-at-its-Core-HIV-Related-Stigma-Across-Contexts.pdf.

Olley, B., S. Seedat and D. Stein. 2004. Self-disclosure of HIV serostatus in recently diagnosed patients with HIV in South Africa. *African Journal of Reproductive Health* 8, 2: 71–6.

Osinde, M., I. Kakaire and D. Kaye. 2012. Factors associated with disclosure of HIV serostatus to sexual partners of patients receiving HIV care in Kabale, Uganda. *International Journal of Gynaecology and Obstetrics* 118, 1: 61–4.

Pan African Christian AIDS Network. 2008. *Situational Analysis: Swaziland Report*. http://www.pacanet.net/index.php?option=com_docman&task=cat_view&gid=23&Itemid=40.

Parker, R. and P. Aggleton. 2003. HIV and AIDS-related stigma and discrimination: A conceptual framework and implications for action. *Social Science & Medicine* 57, 1: 13–24.

Patricks, R. 2000. *Swaziland National Trust Commission*. http://www.sntc.org.sz/cultural/swaziculture4.html#headman.

Piot, P. 2005. Speech given at the London School of Economics London, 8 February. 'Why AIDS is exceptional'. http://www.lse.ac.uk/PublicEvents/pdf/20050208-PiotAIDS2.pdf.

Rapport, N. 2008. Gratuitousness: Notes towards an anthropology of interiority. *Australian Journal of Anthropology* 19, 3: 331–49.

Root, R. 2009. Being positive in church: Religious participation and HIV disclosure rationale among people living with HIV/AIDS in rural Swaziland. *African Journal of AIDS Research* 8, 3: 295–309.

—— 2010. Situating PLWHA experiences of HIV-related stigma in Swaziland. *Global Public Health* 5, 5: 1744–2692.

—— 2011. 'That's when life changed': Church run home-based HIV/AIDS care in Swaziland. A report for the Health Economics and HIV/AIDS Division (HEARD). Durban South Africa: University of KwaZulu-Natal, October 2011.

Root, R. and A. Van Wyngaard. 2011. Free love: A case study of church-run home-based caregivers in a high vulnerability setting. *Global Public Health, Special Supplement: Religious Responses to HIV/AIDS* 6, 2: S174–S191.

Rouleau, G., J. Côté and C. Chantal. 2012. Disclosure experience in a convenience sample of Quebec-born women living with HIV: A phenomenological study. *BMC Women's Health* 12, 1: 37. http://www.biomedcentral.com/1472-6874/12/37.

Ruel, M. 1993. Passages and the person. *Journal of Religion in Africa* 23, 2: 98–124.

Santamaria, E., C. Dolezal, S. Marhefka, S. Hoffman, Y. Ahmed, K. Elkington and C. Mellins. 2011. Psychosocial implications of HIV serostatus disclosure to youth with perinatally acquired HIV. *AIDS Patient Care and STDS* 25, 4: 257–64.

Shamos, S., K. Hartwig and N. Zindela. 2009. Men's and women's experiences with HIV and stigma in Swaziland. *Qualitative Health Research* 19, 12: 1678–89.

Shannon, K., K. Leiter, N. Phaladze, Z. Hlanze, A. Tsai, M. Heisler, V. Iacopino and S. Weiser. 2012. Gender inequity norms are associated with increased male-perpetrated rape and sexual risks for HIV infection in Botswana and Swaziland. *PLoS ONE* 7, 1: e28739. doi:10.1371/journal.pone.0028739.

Simoni, J. and D. Pantalone. 2004. Secrets and safety in the age of AIDS: Does HIV disclosure lead to safer sex? *Topics in HIV Medicine* 12, 4: 109–18.

Singer, M. and S. Clair. 2003. Syndemics and public health: Reconceptualising disease in bio-social context. *Medical Anthropology Quarterly* 17, 4: 423–41.

Skogmar S., D. Shakely, M. Lans, J. Danell, R. Andersson, N. Tshandu, A. Ode'n, S. Roberts and W. Venter. 2006. Effect of antiretroviral treatment and counseling on disclosure of HIV-serostatus in Johannesburg, South Africa. *AIDS Care* 18: 725–30.

Stringer, L., D. Thomas and C. Twyman. 2007. From global politics to local land users: Applying the United Nations convention to combat desertification in Swaziland. *Geographical Journal* 173, 2: 129–42.

Taylor, N. 2006. Working Together? Challenges and Opportunities for International Development Agencies and the Church in the Response to AIDS in Africa. *Tearfund HIV and AIDS Briefing Paper* 7. Middlesex UK: Tearfund.

United Nations Programme on HIV/AIDS (UNAIDS). 2012. *Swaziland. Focus Areas HIV/AIDS.* http://sz.one.un.org/index.php/hiv-and-aids.

UNAIDS Regional Support Team for Eastern and Southern Africa. 2013. *Getting to Zero: HIV in Eastern & Southern Africa.* http://reliefweb.int/sites/reliefweb.int/files/resources/Getting%20to%20Zero.pdf.

United Nations Development Programme. 2008. *Swaziland Human Development Report: HIV and AIDS and culture.* http://hdr.undp.org/en/reports/national/africa/swaziland/name,3316,en.html, accessed 18 November 2013.

United States Department of State. 2008. *Report on International Religious Freedom – Swaziland.* http://www.refworld.org/docid/48d5cbbe8.html.

Vitillo, R. 2009. Faith-based responses to the global HIV pandemic: Exceptional engagement in a major public health emergency. *Journal of Medicine and the Person* 7: 77–84.

Waddell E. and P. Messeri. 2006. Social support, disclosure, and use of antiretroviral therapy. *AIDS and Behavior* 10, 3: 263–72.

Welz, M. 2013. *Integrating Africa: Decolonization's Legacies, Sovereignty and the African Union*. New York: Routledge.

Whiteside, A. and J. Smith. 2009. Exceptional epidemics: AIDS still deserves a global response. *Globalization and Health* 5, 15. doi:10.1186/1744-8603-5-15.

World Bank. 2012. *Swaziland*. http://data.worldbank.org/country/swaziland.

World Health Organization. 2003. Initial steps to developing the World Health Organization's Quality of Life Instrument (WHOQOL) module for international assessment in HIV/AIDS. *AIDS Care* 15, 3: 347–57.

—— 2013. *Swaziland*. http://www.who.int/countries/swz/en/.

Yang, L., A. Kleinman, B. Link, J. Phelan, S. Lee and B. Good. 2007. Culture and stigma: Adding moral experience to stigma theory. *Social Science & Medicine* 64, 7: 1524–35.

Zamberia, A. 2011. HIV-related stigma and access to health care among people living with HIV in Swaziland. *Development Southern Africa* 28, 5: 669–80.

Zwane, P. 2006. Some cultural practices may spread HIV – report. *Swazi Observer* [no month] 19. http://swazilandsolidaritynetworkcanada.wikispaces.com/Some+cultural+practices+may+spread+HIV+-+report.

Chapter 4: Emotional talk

Australian Bureau of Statistics (ABS). 2007. *National Survey of Mental Health and Wellbeing, Summary of Results* (cat. no. 4326.0), released electronically on the ABS website.

Barker, K. 2011. Listening to Lyrica: Contested illnesses and pharmaceutical determinism. *Social Science & Medicine* 73, 6: 833–42.

Blackman, L. 2007. Psychiatric culture and bodies of resistance. *Body and Society* 13, 2: 1–23.

Bos, A. E. R., D. Kanner, O. Muris, B. Janssen and B. Mayer. 2009. Mental illness stigma and disclosure: Consequences of coming out of the closet. *Issues in Mental Health Nursing* 30, 8: 509–13.

Briggs, C. 2007. Anthropology, interviewing, and communicability in contemporary society. *Current Anthropology* 48, 4: 551–80.

Buchbinder, M. 2010. Giving an account of one's pain in the anthropological interview. *Culture, Medicine and Psychiatry* 34, 1: 108–31.

Butler, J. 2005. *Giving an Account of Oneself*. New York: Fordham University Press.

Corrigan, P. W., A. Watson and L. Barr. 2006. The self-stigma of mental illness: Implications for self-esteem and self-efficacy. *Journal of Social and Clinical Psychology* 25, 9: 875–84.

Corrigan, P. W. and A. K. Matthews. 2003. Stigma and disclosure: Implications for coming out of the closet. *Journal of Mental Health* 12, 3: 235–48.

Davidson, J. 2005. Contesting stigma and contested emotions: Personal experience and public perception of specific phobias. *Social Science & Medicine* 61, 10: 2155–64.

Dickson, A., C. Knussen and P. Flowers. 2007. Stigma and the delegitimation experience: An interpretative phenomenological analysis of people living with chronic fatigue syndrome. *Psychology and Health* 22, 7: 851–67.

Dumit, J. 2006. Illnesses you have to fight to get: Facts as forces in uncertain, emergent illnesses. *Social Science & Medicine* 62, 3: 577–90.

Ehrenberg, A. 2010. *The Weariness of the Self: Diagnosing the History of Depression in the Contemporary Age*. London: McGill-Queen's University Press.

Foucault, M. 2001. *Fearless Speech*. Translated and edited by Joseph Pearsons. Los Angeles CA: Semiotext(e).

Fullagar, S. and W. O'Brien. 2012. Immobility, battles and the journey of feeling alive: Women's metaphors of self-transformation through depression and recovery. *Qualitative Health Research* 22, 8: 1063–72.

Jacob, K. 2006. The diagnosis and management of depression and anxiety in primary care: The need for a different framework. *Postgraduate Medical Journal* 82, 974: 836–9.

Jenkins, J. 2011. Pharmaceutical self and imaginary in the social field of psychiatric treatment. In J. Jenkins (ed.) *Pharmaceutical Self: The Global Shaping of Experience in an Age of Psychopharmacology*, pp. 17–40. School of Advanced Research Press.

Koehne, K., B. Hamilton, N. Sands and C. Humpheries. 2012. Working around a contested diagnosis: Borderline personality disorder in adolescence. *Health*, published online 6 June 2012, http://hea.sagepub.com/content/17/1/37.long.

Kokanovic, R., G. Bendelow and B. Philip. 2012. Depression: The ambivalence of diagnosis. *Sociology of Health and Illness* 35, 3: 377–90.

Lafrance, M. 2009. *Women and Depression: Recovery and Resistance*. Routledge: New York.

Leonard, L. and J. M. Ellen. 2008. 'The story of my life': AIDS and 'autobiographical occasions'. *Qualitative Sociology* 31, 1: 37–56.

Manderson, L., E. Bennett and S. Andajani-Sutjahjo. 2006. The social dynamics of the interview: Age, class and gender. *Qualitative Health Research* 16, 10: 1317–34.

Moss, P. and K. Teghtsoonian. 2008. Power and illness: Authority, bodies and context. In P. Moss and K. Teghtsoonian (eds) *Contesting Illness: Processes and Practices*, pp. 3–27. Toronto: University of Toronto Press.

Norman, R. M. G., D. Windell and R. Manchanda. 2010. Examining differences in the stigma of depression and schizophrenia. *International Journal of Social Psychiatry* 58, 1: 69–78.

Pilgrim, D. 2007. The survival of psychiatric diagnosis. *Social Science & Medicine* 65, 3: 536–47.

Pollack, K. 2007. Maintaining face in the presentation of depression: Constraining the therapeutic potential of the consultation. *Health* 11, 2: 163–80.

Ridge, D. and S. Ziebland. 2012. Understanding depression through a 'coming out' framework. *Sociology of Health and Illness* 34, 5: 730–45.

Rogers, A., C. May and D. Oliver. 2001. Experiencing depression, experiencing the depressed: The separate worlds of patients and doctors. *Journal of Mental Health* 10, 3: 317–33.

Scambler, G. 2004. Re-framing stigma: Felt and enacted stigma and challenges to the sociology of chronic and disabling conditions. *Social Theory and Health* 2, 1: 29–46.

Silva, Jennifer M. 2012. Constructing adulthood in an age of uncertainty. *American Sociological Review* 77, 4: 505–22.

Spitzer, R. 2007. Foreword. In A. Horwitz and J. Wakefield (eds) *The Loss of Sadness: How Psychiatry Transformed Normal Sorrow into Depressive Disorder*, pp. vii–x. New York: Oxford University Press.

Whooley, O. 2010. Diagnostic ambivalence: Psychiatric workarounds and the Diagnostic and Statistical Manual of Mental Disorders. *Sociology of Health and Illness* 32, 3: 452–69.

World Health Organization (WHO). 2008. *WHO Global Burden of Disease: 2004 update.* http://www.who.int/healthinfo/global_burden_disease/2004_report_update/en

Chapter 5: HIV/STI prevention technologies and 'strategic (in)visibilities'

Adam, B. 2004. *Intimate confessions.* http://www.hivplusmag.com.

——— 2005. Constructing the neoliberal sexual actor: Responsibility and care of the self in the discourse of barebackers. *Culture, Health and Sexuality* 7, 4: 333–46.

Adam, B., J. Murray, S. Ross, J. Oliver, S. Lincoln and V. Rynard. 2011. hivstigma.com, an innovative web-supported stigma reduction intervention for gay and bisexual men. *Health Education Research* 26, 5: 795–807.

Armstrong, D. 1995. The rise of surveillance medicine. *Sociology of Health and Illness* 17, 3: 393–404.

Aronowitz, R. A. 2009. The converged experience of risk and disease. *Milbank Quarterly* 87, 2: 417–42.

BBC News. 2009. *Pandemic flu service to go live*, Vol. 2012. http://news.bbc.co.uk/2/hi/health/8159316.stm, published online 20 July 2009.

Ben-Ze'ev, A. 2004. *Love Online: Emotions on the Internet.* Cambridge UK: Cambridge University Press.

Blackman, L. 2010. Bodily integrity. *Body & Society* 16, 3: 1–9.

Bond, V. 2010. 'It is not an easy decision on HIV, especially in Zambia': Opting for silence, limited disclosure and implicit understanding to retain a wider identity. *AIDS Care* 22, Suppl. 1: 6–13.

Butler, D. and D. Smith. 2007. Serosorting can potentially increase HIV transmissions. *AIDS* 21, 9: 1218–20.

Cleland, J., J. Caldow and D. Ryan. 2007. A qualitative study of the attitudes of patients and staff to the use of mobile phone technology for recording and gathering asthma data. *Journal of Telemedicine and Telecare* 13, 2: 85–9.

Conrad, P. and V. Leiter. 2004. Medicalisation, markets and consumers. *Journal of Health and Social Behaviour* 45: 158–76.

Cooper, A. and E. Griffin-Shelley. 2002. Introduction. The Internet: The next sexual revolution. In A. Cooper, (ed.) *Sex and the Internet: A Guidebook for Clinicians*, pp. 1–15. New York: Brunner-Routledge.

Davis, M. 2007. Identity, expertise and HIV risk in a case study of reflexivity and medical technologies. *Sociology* 41, 6: 1003–19.

——— 2008. The 'loss of community' and other problems for sexual citizenship in recent HIV prevention. *Sociology of Health and Illness* 30, 2: 182–96.

——— 2009. *Sex, Technology and Public Health.* Houndmills UK: Palgrave.

Davis, M., G. Hart, J. Imrie, O. Davidson, I. Williams and J. Stephenson. 2002. 'HIV is HIV to me': Meanings of treatments, viral load and reinfection among gay men with HIV. *Health, Risk and Society* 4, 1: 31–43.

Davis, M., G. Hart, G. Bolding, L. Sherr and J. Elford. 2006a. E-dating, identity and HIV prevention: Theorising sexualities, risk and network society. *Sociology of Health & Illness* 28, 4: 457–78.

—— 2006b. Sex and the internet: Gay men, risk reduction and serostatus. *Culture, Health and Sexuality* 8, 2: 161–74.

Emlet, C. 2008. Truth and consequences: A qualitative exploration of HIV disclosure in older adults. *AIDS Care* 20, 6: 710–17.

Eustace, R. and P. Ilagan. 2010. HIV disclosure among HIV positive individuals: A concept analysis. *Journal of Advanced Nursing* 66, 9: 2094–103.

Flowers, P. and M. Davis. 2012. Obstinate essentialism: Managing identity transformations amongst gay men living with HIV. *Psychology & Sexuality*. DOI: 10.1080/19419899.2012.679364.

Flowers, P., D. Langdridge, B. Gough and R. Holliday. In press. On the biomedicalisation of the penis: The commodification of function and aesthetics. *International Journal of Men's Health*.

Flowers, P. and J. Frankis. 2000. Community, responsibility and culpability: HIV risk-management amongst Scottish gay men. *Journal of Community and Applied Social Psychology* 10: 285–300.

Foucault, M. 1978. *The History of Sexuality, Volume 1: An Introduction*. London: Penguin.

—— 1982. *Discipline and Punish: The Birth of the Prison*. Harmondsworth UK: Penguin.

—— 1988. Technologies of the self. In L. Martin, H. Gutman and P. Hutton (eds) *Technologies of the Self: A Seminar with Michel Foucault*, pp. 16–49. Amherst MA: University of Massachusetts Press.

—— 1990. *The Care of the Self: The History of Sexuality*, Volume 3. London: Penguin.

Fox, N. and K. Ward. 2006. Health identities: From expert patient to resisting consumer. *Health: An Interdisciplinary Journal for the Social Study of Health, Illness and Medicine* 10, 4: 461–79.

Frith, L. 2007. HIV self-testing: A time to revise current policy. *The Lancet* 369, 9557: 243–5.

Goffman, E. 1959. *The Presentation of Self in Everyday Life*. Harmondsworth UK: Penguin.

—— 1983. The interaction order. *American Sociological Review* 48: 1–17.

—— 1986 [1963]. *Stigma: Notes on the Management of Spoiled Identity*. Harmondsworth UK: Penguin.

Goss, J. 2008. *Projection of Australian health care expenditure by disease, 2003 to 2033*. Cat. no. HWE 43. Canberra ACT: Australian Institute of Health and Welfare.

Green, G. and E. Sobo. 2000. *The Endangered Self: Managing the Social Risks of HIV*. London: Routledge.

Hartley, H. 2006. The 'pinking' of viagra culture: Drug industry efforts to create and repackage sex drugs for women. *Sexualities* 9, 3: 363–78.

Imrie, J., J. Elford, S. Kippax and G. Hart. 2007. Biomedical HIV prevention and social science. *The Lancet* 370, 7 July: 10–11.

International Association of Physicians in AIDS Care. 2012. *Controlling the HIV epidemic with antiretrovirals: HIV treatment as prevention and pre-exposure prophylaxis: Consensus Statement*, http://www.iapac.org.

Kalichman, S., C. Di Marco, J. Austin, W. Luke and K. Di Fonzo. 2003. Stress, social support, and HIV-status disclosure to family and friends among HIV-positive men and women. *Journal of Behavioral Medicine* 26, 4: 315–32.

Kirby Institute. 2011. HIV, viral hepatitis and sexually transmissable infections in Australia. *Annual Surveillance Report 2011*. Sydney NSW: The Kirby Institute, University of New South Wales.

—— 2012. HIV, viral hepatitis and sexually transmissible infections in Australia. *Annual Surveillance Report 2012*. Sydney NSW: The Kirby Institute, University of NSW.

Klausner, J., W. Wolf, L. Fischer-Ponce, I. Zolt and M. Katz. 2000. Tracing a syphilis outbreak through cyberspace. *Journal of the American Medical Association* 284, 4: 447–9.

Lefebvre, C. 2009. Integrating cell phones and mobile technologies into public health practice: A social marketing perspective. *Health Promotion Practice* 10, 4: 490–4.

Levine, D. and J. Klausner. 2005. Lessons learned from tobacco control: A proposal for public health policy initiatives to reduce the consequences of high-risk sexual behaviour among men who have sex with men and use the internet. *Sexuality Research & Social Policy* 2, 1: 51–8.

Lupton, D. 2000. Foucault and the medicalisation critique. In A. Petersen and R. Bunton (eds) *Foucault, Health and Medicine*. London: Routledge.

Mao, L., J. Crawford, H. Hopsers, G. Prestage, A. Grulich, J. Kaldor and S. Kippax. 2006. 'Serosorting' in casual anal sex of HIV-negative gay men is noteworthy and is increasing in Sydney, Australia. *AIDS* 20, 8: 1204–6.

Mayfield Arnold, E., E. Rice, D. Flannery and M. Rotheram-Borus. 2008. HIV disclosure among adults living with HIV. *AIDS Care* 20, 1: 80–92.

Mead, G. 1913. The social self. *Journal of Philosophy, Psychology and Scientific Methods* 10, 14: 374–80.

National Health and Medical Research Council. 2008. http://www.nhmrc.gov.au/your-health/egenetics/direct-consumer-dtc-dna-tests.

Persson, A. and W. Richards. 2008. From closet to heterotopia: A conceptual exploration of disclosure and 'passing' among heterosexuals living with HIV. *Culture, Health & Sexuality* 10, 1: 73–86.

Petersen, A. and D. Lupton. 1996. *The New Public Health: Health and Self in the Age of Risk*. St Leonards NSW: Allen & Unwin.

Race, K. 2010. Click here for HIV status: Shifting templates of sexual negotiation. *Emotion, Space and Society* 3: 7–14.

Ross, M., B. Rosser, E. Coleman and R. Mazin. 2006. Misrepresentation on the internet and in real life about sex and HIV: A study of Latino men who have sex with men. *Culture, Health & Sexuality* 8, 2: 133–44.

Serovich, J. 2001. A test of two HIV disclosure theories. *AIDS Education and Prevention* 13, 4: 355–64.

Serovich, J., Y. J. Lim and T. M. Mason. 2008. A retest of two HIV disclosure theories: The women's story. *Health and Social Work* 33, 1: 23–31.

Sowell, R. L., B. F. Seals, K. D. Phillips and C. H. Julious. 2003. Disclosure of HIV infection: How do women decide to tell? *Health Education Research* 18, 1: 32–44.

Squire, C. 2007. *HIV in South Africa: Talking about the Big Thing*. London: Routledge.

Webster, A. 2007. *Health, Technology & Society: A Sociological Critique*. Houndmills UK: Palgrave.

Whitty, M. and A. Carr. 2006. *Cyberspace Romance: The Psychology of Online Relationships.* Houndmills UK: Palgrave Macmillan.

World Health Organization. 2010. *Developing Sexual Health Programmes: A Framework for Action.* Geneva: Department of Reproductive Health and Research, World Health Organization.

Chapter 6: Is it 'disclosure'?

Ablon, J. 1992. Social dimensions of genetic disorders. *Practicing Anthropology* 14, 1: 10–13.

Almqvist, E. W., M. Bloch, R. Brinkman, D. Craufurd and M. R. Hayden. 1999. A worldwide assessment of the frequency of suicide, suicide attempts, or psychiatric hospitalization after predictive testing for Huntington disease. *American Journal of Human Genetics* 64, 5: 1293–304.

Barclay, L. A. and K. S. Markel. 2007. Discrimination and stigmatisation in work organisations: A multiple level framework for research on genetic testing. *Human Relations* 60, 6: 953–80.

Biesecker, B. 1998. Future directions in genetic counseling: Practical and ethical considerations. *Kennedy Institute of Ethics Journal* 8, 2: 145–60.

Billings, P. R., M. A. Kohn, M. de Cuevas, J. S. Alper and M. R. Natowicz. 1992. Discrimination as a consequence of genetic testing. *American Journal of Human Genetics* 50, 3: 476–82.

Bloch, M., S. Adam, S. Wiggins, M. Huggins and M. R. Hayden. 2005. Predictive testing for Huntington disease in Canada: The experience of those receiving an increased risk. *American Journal of Medical Genetics* 42, 4: 499–507.

Browner, C. H. and N. Press. 1996. The production of authoritative knowledge in American prenatal care. *Medical Anthropology Quarterly* 10, 2: 141–56.

Browner, C. H. and H. M. Preloran. 2010. *Neurogenetic Diagnoses: The Power of Hope and the Limits of Today's Medicine.* New York: Routledge.

Burgess, M. M. and L. d'Agincourt-Canning. 2001. Genetic testing for hereditary disease: Attending to relational responsibility. *Journal of Clinical Ethics* 12, 4: 361–72.

Burke, W., L. E. Pinsky and N. A. Press. 2003. Categorizing genetic tests to identify their ethical, legal, and social implications. *American Journal of Medical Genetics* 106, 3: 233–40.

Chapman, M. A. 2005. Canadian experience with predictive testing for Huntington disease: Lessons for genetic testing centers and policy makers. *American Journal of Medical Genetics* 42, 4: 491–8.

Chapple, A., C. May and P. Campion. 1995. Lay understanding of genetic disease: A British study of families attending a genetic counseling service. *Journal of Genetic Counseling* 4, 4: 281–300.

Claes, E., G. Evers-Kiebooms, A. Boogaerts, M. Decruyenaere, L. Denayer and E. Legius. 2002. Communication with close and distant relatives in the context of genetic testing for hereditary breast and ovarian cancer in cancer patients. *American Journal of Medical Genetics* Part A 116, 1: 11–19.

Coleman, M., J. Troilo and T. Jamison. 1996. The diversity of stepmothers: The influences of stigma, gender, and context on stepmother identities. In J. Pryor (ed.) *The International Handbook of Stepfamilies: Policy and Practice in Legal, Research, and Clinical Environments*, pp. 369–93. Hoboken NJ: John Wiley & Sons.

Cox, S. M. and W. McKellin. 2001. 'There's this thing in our family': Predictive testing and the construction of risk for Huntington disease. *Sociology of Health & Illness* 21, 5: 622–46.

Crocker, J., B. Major and C. L. Steele. 1998. Social stigma. In D. T. Gilbert, S. T. Fiske and G. Lindzey (eds) *The Handbook of Social Psychology*, pp. 504–53. New York: Oxford University Press.

Crocker, J. and J. A. Garcia. 2006. Stigma and the social basis of the self: A synthesis. In S. Levin and C. van Laar (eds) *Stigma and Group Inequality: Social Psychological Perspectives*, pp. 287–308. Mahwah NJ: Lawrence Erlbaum Associates.

Etchegary, H. 2006. Genetic testing for Huntington's disease: How is the decision taken? *Genetic Testing* 10, 1: 60–7.

Evers-Kiebooms, G., M. Welkenhuysen, E. Claes, M. Ducruyenaere and L. Denayer. 2000. The psychological complexity of predictive testing for late onset neurogenetic diseases and hereditary cancers: Implications for multidisciplinary counseling and for genetic education. *Social Science & Medicine* 51, 6: 831–41.

Featherstone, K., P. Atkinson, A. Bharadwaj and A. Clarke. 2006. *Risky Relations: Family, Kinship and the New Genetics*. Oxford UK: Berg Publishers.

Finkler, K. 2000. *Experiencing the New Genetics: Family and Kinship on the Medical Frontier*. Philadelphia PA: University of Pennsylvania Press.

Flowers, P., M. Davis, G. Hart, M. Rosengarten, J. Frankis and J. Imrie. 2006. Diagnosis and stigma and identity amongst HIV positive Black Africans living in the UK. *Psychology and Health* 21, 1: 109–22.

Forrest, K., S. A. Simpson, B. J. Wilson, E. R. can Teijlingen, L. McKee, N. Haites and E. Matthews. 2003. To tell or not to tell: Barriers and facilitators in family communication about genetic risk. *Clinical Genetics* 64, 4: 317–26.

Goffman, E. 1963. *Stigma: Notes on the Management of Spoiled Identity*. New York: Simon & Schuster.

Greely, H. T. 2005. Banning genetic discrimination. *New England Journal of Medicine* 353, 9: 865–7.

Hallowell, N. 1999. Doing the right thing: Genetic risk and responsibility. *Sociology of Health & Illness* 21, 5: 597–621.

Hallowell, N., C. Foster, R. Eeles, A. Ardern-Jones, V. Murday and M. Watson. 2003. Balancing autonomy and responsibility: The ethics of generating and disclosing genetic information. *Journal of Medical Ethics* 29, 2: 74–9.

Henneman, L., L. Kooij, K. Bouman and L. P. ten Kate. 2002. Personal experiences of cystic fibrosis (CF) carrier couples prospectively identified in CF families. *American Journal of Medical Genetics* 110, 4: 324–31.

Herdt, G. 2001. Stigma and the ethnographic study of HIV: Problems and prospects. *AIDS and Behavior* 5, 2: 141–9.

Hess, P. G., H. M. Preloran and C. H. Browner. 2009. Diagnostic genetic testing for a fatal illness: The experience of patients with movement disorders. *New Genetics and Society* 28, 1: 3–18.

Hudson, K. L. 2007. Prohibiting genetic discrimination. *New England Journal of Medicine* 356, 20: 2021–3.

Hudson, K. L., M. K. Holohan and F. S. Collins. 2008. Keeping pace with the times: The Genetic Information Nondiscrimination Act of 2008. *New England Journal of Medicine* 358, 25: 2661–3.

Huggins, M., M. Bloch, S. Wiggins, S. Adam, O. Suchowersky, M. Trew and M. Kimek. 2005. Predictive testing for Huntington disease in Canada: Adverse effects and unexpected results in those receiving a decreased risk. *American Journal of Medical Genetics* 42, 4: 508–15.

Hunt, L. M., C. H. Browner and B. Jordan. 1990. Hypoglycemia: Portrait of an illness construct in everyday use. *Medical Anthropology Quarterly* 4, 2: 191–210.

Jones, E. E., A. Farou, A. H. Hasdorf, H. Markus, D. T. Miller and R. A. Scott. 1984. *Social Stigma: The Psychology of Marked Relationships*. New York: W. H. Freeman.

Kenen, R. H. 1994. The Human Genome Project: Creator of the potentially sick, potentially vulnerable and potentially stigmatized? In I. Robinson (ed.) *Life and Death under High Technology Medicine*, pp. 49–64. Manchester UK: Manchester University Press.

Klitzman, R., D. Thorne, J. Williamson, W. Chung and K. Marder. 2007. Disclosures of Huntington disease risk within families: Patterns of decision-making and implications. *American Journal of Medical Genetics* Part A 143, 16: 1835–49.

Koenig, B. A. and A. Stockdale. 2011. The promise of molecular medicine in preventing disease: Examining the burden of genetic risk. In D. Callahan (ed.) *Promoting Healthy Behavior: How much Freedom? Whose Responsibility?*, pp. 116–37. Washington DC: Georgetown University Press.

Konrad, M. 2005. *Narrating the New Predictive Genetics: Ethics, Ethnography, and Science*. Cambridge UK: Cambridge University Press.

Lehmann, L. S., J. C. Weeks, N. Klar, L. Biener and J. E. Garber. 2000. Disclosure of familial genetic information: Perceptions of the duty to inform. *American Journal of Medicine* 109, 9: 705–11.

Link, B. G. and J. C. Phelan. 2001. Conceptualizing stigma. *Annual Review of Sociology* 27: 363–85.

Major, B. and L. T. O'Brien. 2005. The social psychology of stigma. *Annual Review of Psychology* 56: 393–421.

Meiser, B. and S. Dunn. 2000. Psychological impact of genetic testing for Huntington's disease: An update of the literature. *Journal of Neurology, Neurosurgery & Psychiatry* 69, 5: 574–8.

Meiser, B., P. B. Mitchell, H. McGirr, M. Van Herten and P. R. Schofield. 2005. Implications of genetic risk information in families with a high density of bipolar disorder: An exploratory study. *Social Science & Medicine* 60, 1: 109–18.

Opala, J. and F. Boillot. 1996. Leprosy among the Limba: Illness and healing in the context of world view. *Social Science & Medicine* 42, 1: 3–19.

Ormond, K. E., P. L. Mills, L. A. Lester and L. F. Ross. 2003. Effect of family history on disclosure patterns of cystic fibrosis carrier status. *American Journal of Medical Genetics, Part C: Seminars in Medical Genetics* 119C, 1: 70–7.

Oyserman, D. and J. K. Swim. 2002. Stigma: An insider's view. *Journal of Social Issues* 57, 1: 1–14.

Parker, R. and P. Aggleton. 2003. HIV and AIDS-related stigma and discrimination: A conceptual framework and implications for action. *Social Science & Medicine* 57, 1: 13–24.

Pembrey, M. 1996. The new genetics: A user's guide. In T. Marteau and M. Richards (eds) *The Troubled Helix: Social and Psychological Implications of the New Human Genetics*, pp. 63–81. Cambridge UK: Cambridge University Press.

Petersen, A. 2006. The best experts: The narratives of those who have a genetic condition. *Social Science & Medicine* 63, 1: 32–42.

Quinn, D. M. 2006. Concealable versus conspicuous stigmatised identities. In S. Levin and C. Van Laar (eds) *Stigma and Group Inequality: Social Psychological Perspectives*, pp. 83–103. Mahwah NJ: Lawrence Erlbaum Associates.

Rabinow, P. 1992. From sociobiology to biosociality: Artificiality and enlightenment. In *Zone 6: Incorporations*, pp. 91–111 New York: Zone Books.

Sankar, P., M. K. Cho, P. R. Wolpe and C. Shairer. 2006. What is in a cause? Exploring the relationship between genetic cause and felt stigma. *Genetics in Medicine* 8, 1: 33–42.

Sayce, L. 1998. Stigma, discrimination and social exclusion: What's in a word? *Journal of Mental Health* 7, 4: 331–43.

Sharpe, N. F., R. F. Carter, N. P. Callanan and B. S. Leroy. 2006. Genetic counseling and the physician–patient relationship. In N. F. Sharpe and R. F. Carter (eds) *Genetic Testing: Care, Consent, and Liability*, pp. 1–23. Hoboken NJ: Wiley.

Shuttleworth, R. P. and D. Kasnitz. 2004. Stigma, community, ethnography: Joan Ablon's contribution to the anthropology of impairment-disability. *Medical Anthropology Quarterly* 18, 2: 139–61.

Smith, K. R., C. D. Zick, R. N. Mayer and J. R. Botkin. 2002. Voluntary disclosure of BRCA1 mutation test results. *Genetic Testing* 6, 2: 89–92.

Vernon, M. 2012. 'Not just a guy in a dress': Transsexual Embodiment, Identity, and Genital Reassignment Surgery in the U.S. PhD dissertation, Department of Anthropology, University of California, Los Angeles.

Yang, L. H., A. Kleinman, B. G. Link, J. C. Phelan, S. Lee and B. Good. 2007. Culture and stigma: Adding moral experience to stigma theory. *Social Science & Medicine* 64, 7: 1524–35.

Chapter 7: Disclosure as method, disclosure as dilemma

Auerbach, E. 2003 [1953]. *Mimesis: The Representation of Reality in Western Literature*. Transl. W. R. Trask. Princeton NJ: Princeton University Press.

Behar, R. 2003 [1994]. *Translated Woman: Crossing the Border with Esperanza's Story*. New York: Beacon Books.

Biehl, J. 2005. *Vita: Life in a Zone of Social Abandonment*. Berkeley CA: University of California Press.

Bourgois, P. and J. Schonberg. 2009. *Righteous Dopefiend*. Berkeley CA: University of California Press.

Brettell, C. (ed.). 1996. *When They Read What We Write: The Politics of Ethnography*. Westport CT: Praeger.

Briggs, J. 1971. *Never in Anger: Portrait of an Eskimo Family*. Cambridge MA: Harvard University Press.

Cannell, F. 2005. The Christianity of anthropology. *Journal of the Royal Anthropological Institute* 11, 2: 335–6.

Clifford, J. and G. Marcus (eds). 1986. *Writing Culture: The Poetics and Politics of Ethnography*. Berkeley CA: University of California Press.

Das, V. 2006. *Life and Words: Violence and the Descent into the Ordinary*. Berkeley CA: University of California Press.

Evans-Pritchard, E. E. 1940. *The Nuer*. London: Oxford University.

Faubion, J. D. 2011. *An Anthropology of Ethics*. New York: Cambridge University Press.

Favret-Saada, J. 1981. *Deadly Words: Witchcraft in the Bocage*. New York: Cambridge University Press.

Haraway, D. 1997. *Modest_Witness@Second_Millennium.FemaleMan(©_Meets_ OncoMouse^{TM}*. New York: Routledge.

Helmreich, S. 2009. *Alien Ocean: Anthropological Voyages in Microbial Seas*. Berkeley CA: University of California Press.

Hymes, D. (ed.). 1974. *Reinventing Anthropology*. New York: Vintage Books.

Iser, W. 1978. *The Act of Reading: A Theory of Aesthetic Response*. Baltimore MD: Johns Hopkins University Press.

Jameson, Fredric. 1991. *Postmodernism, or, The Cultural Logic of Late Capitalism*. Durham NC: Duke University Press.

Marcus, G. E. and M. M. J. Fischer. 1986. *Anthropology as Cultural Critique: An Experimental Moment in the Human Sciences*. Chicago IL: University of Chicago Press.

Martin, E. 2007. *Bipolar Expeditions: Mania and Depression in American Culture*. Princeton NJ: Princeton University Press.

McLuhan, M. 1994 [1964]. *Understanding Media: The Extensions of Man*. Cambridge MA: MIT Press.

Priest, C. 1996 [1981]. *The Affirmation*. London: Simon & Schuster.

Shapin, S. and S. Schaffer. 1989. *Leviathan and the Air-pump*. Princeton NJ: Princeton University Press.

Suvin, D. 1979. *Metamorphoses of Science Fiction: On the Poetics and History of a Literary Genre*. New Haven CT: Yale University Press.

Taussig, M. 1997. *The Magic of the State*. New York: Routledge.

Wolf-Meyer, M. 2008. Sleep, signification, and the abstract body of allopathic medicine. *Body & Society* 14, 4: 93–114.

—— 2009. Precipitating pharmakologies and capital entrapments: Narcolepsy and the strange cases of Provigil and Xyrem. *Medical Anthropology: Cross-Cultural Studies in Health and Illness* 28, 1: 11–30.

—— 2011. The nature of sleep. *Comparative Studies in Society and History* 53, 4: 945–70.

—— 2012. *The Slumbering Masses: Sleep, Medicine, and Modern American Life*. Minneapolis MN: University of Minnesota Press.

—— 2014. Therapy, remedy, cure: Disorder and the spatiotemporality of medicine and everyday life. *Medical Anthropology* [in press].

Chapter 8: Transsexual women's strategies of disclosure and social geographies of knowledge

Beauchamp, T. 2009. Artful concealment and strategic visibility: Transgender bodies and U.S. state surveillance after 9/11. *Surveillance and Society* 6, 4: 356–66.

de Beauvoir, S. 1961. *The Second Sex*. New York: Bantam

Benjamin, H. 1966. *The Transsexual Phenomenon*. New York: Julian Press.

Bettcher, T. 2007. Evil deceivers and make-believers: On transphobic violence and the politics of illusion. *Hypatia* 22, 3: 43–65.

—— 2012. Full frontal morality: The naked truth about gender. *Hypatia* 27, 2: 19–37.

Bruner, J. 1997. The narrative model of self construction. In R. L. Thompson (ed.) *The Self Across Psychology: Self-recognition, Self-awareness, and the Self-concept*, pp. 145–61. New York: New York Academy of Science.

Connell, C. 2010. Doing, undoing, or redoing gender? Learning from the workplace experiences of transpeople. *Gender and Society* 24, 1: 31–55.

Davis, E. 2008. Situating fluidity: (Trans) gender identification and the regulation of gender diversity. *GLQ* 15, 1: 97–130.

Garfinkel, H. 1967. *Studies in Ethnomethodology*. Englewood Cliffs NJ: Prentice-Hall.

Gergen, K. and M. Gergen. 1983. Narratives of the self. In T. R. Sarbin and K. E. Scheibe (eds) *Studies of Social Identity*, pp. 254–73. New York: Praeger.

Green, R. and J. Money (eds). 1969 *Transsexualism and Sex Reassignment*. Baltimore MD: Johns Hopkins Press.

Kleinman, A. 1999. Moral experience and ethical reflection: Can ethnography reconcile them? A quandary for 'the new bioethics'. *Daedalus* 128, 4: 69–97.

Kosenko, K. 2010. Meanings and dilemmas of sexual safety and communication for transgender individuals. *Health Communication* 25, 2: 131–41.

Marshall, P. 1992. Anthropology and bioethics. *Medical Anthropology Quarterly* 6, 1: 49–73.

Mason-Schrock, D. 1996. Transsexual narrative construction of the self. *Social Psychology Quarterly* 59, 3: 176–92.

Meyerowitz, J. 2002. *How Sex Changed: A History of Transsexuality in the United States*. Cambridge MA: Harvard University Press.

Muller, J. 1994. Anthropology, bioethics, and medicine: A provocative trilogy. *Medical Anthropology Quarterly* 8, 4: 448–67.

Reed, N. 2012. The 'ethical imperative' of disclosure, or: How to believe your victim owes you an opportunity for abuse. http://freethoughtblogs.com/natalie reed/2012/03/20/the-ethical-imperative-of-disclosure-or-how-to-believe-your-victim-owes-you-an-opportunity-for-abuse/.

Robbins, J. 2007. Between reproduction and freedom: Morality, value and radical change. *Ethnos: Journal of Anthropology* 72, 3: 293–314.

—— 2009. Value, structure, and the range of possibilities. *Ethnos: Journal of Anthropology* 74, 2: 277–85.

Ruby, J. and K. Mantilla. 2000. Men in ewes' clothing: The stealth politics of the transgender movement. *Off Our Backs* 30, 4: 5–12.

Schrock, D. and L. Reid. 2006. Transsexuals' sexual stories. *Archives of Sexual Behavior* 35, 1: 75–86.

Sharpe, A. 2012. Transgender and the legal obligation to disclose gender history. *Modern Law Review* 75, 1: 33–53.

Sobo, E. 1997. Self-disclosure and self-construction among HIV positive people: The rhetorical uses of stereotypes and sex. *Anthropology and Medicine* 4, 1: 67–87.

Stone, S. 1991. The empire strikes back: A posttranssexual manifesto. In J. Epstein and K. Straub (eds) *Body Guards: The Cultural Politics of Gender Ambiguity*, pp. 280–304. New York: Routledge.

Turner, L. 2003a. Bioethics in multicultural world: Medicine and morality in pluralistic settings. *Health Care Analysis* 11, 2: 99–117.

—— 2003b. Zones of consensus and zones of conflict: Questioning the 'common morality' presumption in bioethics. *Kennedy Institute of Ethics Journal* 13, 3: 193–218.

Vernon, M. 2012. 'Not just a guy in a dress': Transsexual identity, embodiment, and genital reassignment surgery in the United States. PhD Dissertation, Department of Anthropology, University of California, Los Angeles.

Zigon, J. 2007. Moral breakdown and the ethical demand: A theoretical framework for an anthropology of moralities. *Anthropological Theory* 7, 2: 131–50.
—— 2009. Within a range of possibilities: Morality and ethics in social life. *Ethnos: Journal of Anthropology* 74, 2: 251–76.

Chapter 9: HIV disclosure

Andrews, M., C. Squire and M. Tamboukou (eds). 2013. *Doing Narrative Research*, 2nd edn. London: Sage Publications.
Bernays, S., T. Rhodes and A. Prodanovic. 2007. *HIV Treatment Access, Delivery and Uncertainty: A Qualitative Study in Serbia and in Montenegro*. London: London School of Hygiene and Tropical Medicine/UNDP.
Beverley, J. 2004. *Testimonio: On the Politics of Truth*. Minneapolis MN: University of Minnesota Press.
Butler, J. 2005. *Giving an Account of Oneself*. Bronx NY: Fordham University Press.
Campbell, C., Y. Nair, S. Maimane and J. Nicholson. 2007. 'Dying twice': A multi-level model of the roots of AIDS stigma in two South African communities. *Journal of Health Psychology* 12, 3: 403–16.
Cohen, M., Y. Chen, M. McCauley, T. Gamble, M. Hosseinipour et al. 2011. Prevention of HIV-1 infection with early antiretroviral therapy. *New England Journal of Medicine* 365, 6: 493–505.
Crimp, D. (ed.). 1988. *AIDS: Cultural Analysis/Cultural Activism*. Boston MA: MIT Press.
Davis, M. and C. Squire. 2010. HIV technologies. In M. Davis and C. Squire (eds) *HIV Treatment and Prevention Technologies in International Perspective*, pp. 1–17. London: Palgrave Macmillan.
Davis, M. and P. Flowers. 2011. Love and HIV serodiscordance in gay men's accounts of life with their regular partners. *Culture, Health and Sexuality* 13, 7: 737–49.
Derrida, J. 2001. *A Taste for the Secret*. London: Polity Press.
Elliott, J. 2013. Suffering agency: Imagining neoliberal personhood in North America and Britain. *Social Text* 31, 2: 83–101.
Foucault, M. 1975. *Discipline and Punish*. New York: Random House.
—— 1991. Governmentality. In G. Burchell, C. Gordon and P. Miller (eds) *The Foucault Effect: Studies in Governmentality*, pp. 87–104. Hemel Hempstead: Harvester Wheatsheaf.
—— 1997. *The Politics of Truth*. New York: Semiotext(e)
Friedman, E. and Squire, C. 1998. *Morality USA*. Minneapolis MN: Minnesota University Press.
Health Protection Agency. 2011. *HIV in the UK: 2011 Report*. London: Health Protection Services, Colindale.
—— 2012. *HIV in the UK: 2012 Report*. London: Health Protection Services, Colindale.
Heywood, M. 2009. *South Africa's Treatment Action Campaign: Combining law and social mobilisation to realise the right to health*. http://www.section27.org.za/wp-content/uploads/2010/04/journal-HR-practice-heywood.pdf Accessed 24.05.2013.
Iwelunmor, J., N. Zungu and C. Airhihenbuwa. 2010. Rethinking HIV disclosure among women within the context of motherhood in South Africa. *American Journal of Public Health* 100, 8: 1393–9.

Joffe, H. 2006. Anxiety, mass crisis and 'the other'. In P. 6, S. Radstone, C. Squire and A. Treacher (eds) *Public Emotions*, pp. 161–80. London: Palgrave Macmillan.

Kvale, S. 2008. *InterViews*. London: Sage Publications.

MacIntyre, A. 1984. *After Virtue*. Notre Dame IN: Notre Dame University Press.

Mbali, M. 2005. *TAC in the history of rights-based, patient driven HIV/AIDS activism in South Africa.* http://quod.lib.umich.edu/p/passages/4761530.0010.011?rgn=main;view=fulltext.

National AIDS Trust. 2011. *Fluctuating Symptoms of HIV*. London: National AIDS Trust.

Nguyen, V.-K. 2010. *The Republic of Therapy*. Chapel Hill NC: Duke University Press.

Ong, A. 2006. *Neoliberalism as Exception*. Chapel Hill NC: Duke University Press.

Riessman, C. 2008. *Narrative Methods for the Human Sciences*. Thousand Oaks CA: Sage Publications

Robins, S. 2009. *From Revolution to Rights in South Africa*. Oxford UK: James Currey, with University of KwaZulu-Natal Press.

Rose, N. 1990. *Governing the Soul*. London: Routledge.

—— 2007. *The Politics of Life Itself*. Princeton NJ: Princeton University Press.

Sontag, S. 1989. *AIDS and Its Metaphors*. New York: Farrar, Straus & Giroux.

Squire, C. 1999. 'Neighbors who might become friends': Selves, genres and citizenship in stories of HIV. *Sociological Quarterly* 40, 11: 109–37.

—— 2003. Can an HIV positive woman find true love? Romance in the stories of women living with HIV. *Feminism and Psychology* 13, 1: 73–100.

—— 2006. Feeling entitled: HIV, entitlement feelings and citizenship. In P. 6, S. Radstone, C. Squire and A. Treacher (eds) *Public Emotions*, pp. 202–30. London: Palgrave Macmillan.

—— 2012. *What is Narrative? NCRM Working Paper*. http://eprints.ncrm.ac.uk/3065/.

—— 2013. *Living with HIV and ARVs: Three Letter Lives*. London: Palgrave Macmillan.

Treichler, P. 1999. *How to Have Theory in an Epidemic*. Chapel Hill NC: Duke University Press.

UNAIDS. 2012. *Global Report: UNAIDS Report on the Global HIV Epidemic*. Geneva: UNAIDS.

Watney, S. 1994. *Practices of Freedom*. Chapel Hill NC: Duke University Press.

Chapter 10: Contours of truth

Altman, D. 2013. *The End of the Homosexual?* St Lucia QLD: University of Queensland Press.

Bauman, Z. 2003. *Liquid Love: On the Frailty of Human Bonds*. Cambridge UK: Polity.

Beck, U. and E. Beck-Gernsheim. 1995. *The Normal Chaos of Love*. Cambridge UK: Polity.

Butler, J. 2005. *Giving an Account of Oneself*. New York: Fordham University Press.

Clarke, A., L. Mamo, J. Fosket, J. Fishman and J. Shim (eds). 2010. *Biomedicalization: Technoscience, Health, and Illness in the U.S.* Durham NC: Duke University Press.

Dyson, S., K. Atkin, L. Culley, S. Dyson, H. Evans and D. Rowley. 2010. Disclosure and sickle cell disorder: A mixed methods study of the young person with sickle cell at school. *Social Science & Medicine* 70, 12: 2036–44.

Foucault, M. 1982. *Discipline and Punish: The Birth of the Prison*. Harmondsworth UK: Penguin.

—— 1988. Technologies of the self. In L. Martin, H. Gutman, and P. Hutton (eds) *Technologies of the Self: A Seminar with Michel Foucault*, pp. 16–49. Amherst MA: University of Massachusetts Press.

Frank, A. 1995. *The Wounded Storyteller: Body, Illness and Ethics*. Chicago IL: University of Chicago Press.

Freud, S. 1962 [1927]. *The Ego and the Id*. London: Hogarth Press.

Goffman, E. 1959. *The Presentation of Self in Everyday Life*. Harmondsworth UK: Penguin.

—— 1963. *Stigma: Notes on the Management of Spoiled Identity*. Harmondsworth UK: Penguin.

Irvine, A. 2011. Something to declare? The disclosure of common mental health problems at work. *Disability & Society* 26, 2: 179–92.

Kairania, R., R. Gray, N. Kiwanuka, F. Makumbi, N. Sewankambo, D. Serwadda, F. Nalugoda, G. Kigozi, J. Semanda and M. Wawer. 2010. Disclosure of HIV results among discordant couples in Rakai, Uganda: A facilitated couple counselling approach. *AIDS Care: Psychological and Socio-medical Aspects of AIDS/ HIV* 22, 9: 1041–51.

Kirkova, D. 2013. 'I look back and I can't believe the strength he had': Catherine Zeta Jones opens up about her husband's battle with cancer, and her own wrestle with bipolar disorder. *Daily Mail Online*. http://www.dailymail.co.uk/femail/ article-2372304/Catherine-Zeta-Jones-bipolar-disorder-husband-Michael-Douglas-cancer-battle.html.

Mauss, M. 1990 [1950]. *The Gift: The Form and Reason for Exchange in Archaic Societies*. London: Routledge.

Mead, G. 1913. The social self. *Journal of Philosophy, Psychology and Scientific Methods* 10, 14: 374–80.

Payne, E. 2013. Angelina Jolie undergoes double mastectomy. *CNN* (online edition). http://edition.cnn.com/2013/05/14/showbiz/angelina-jolie-double-mastectomy.

Plummer, K. 1995. *Telling Sexual Stories: Power, Change and Social Worlds*. London: Routledge.

—— 2003. *Intimate Citizenship: Private Decisions and Public Dialogues*. Seattle WA: University of Washington Press.

Rayner, G. 2013. Stephen Fry: I attempted to kill myself in 2012. *The Telegraph* (online edition). http://www.telegraph.co.uk/news/celebritynews/10102024/ Stephen-Fry-I-attempted-to-kill-myself-in-2012.html.

Suthers, G,. E. McCusker and S. Wake. 2011. Alerting genetic relatives to a risk of serious inherited disease without a patient's consent. *Medical Journal Australia* 194, 8: 385–6.

Index

Milton Keynes UK
Ingram Content Group UK Ltd.
UKHW031537071024
449327UK00024B/1859